Type 2 Diabetes Cookbook
Beginner's Quick & Easy Recipes for Delicious Diabetes Diets

300 Healthy

Lunches

for

Diabetic Wellness in 30 Minutes or Less

By

Lily Anders

Copyright Page

Ace East Publishing LLC
1401 21st Street
Suite R
Sacramento, CA 95811

ISBN: **978-1-963939-85-9**

First Edition

ACE EAST
PUBLISHING

Disclaimer Page

This cookbook is crafted to offer insightful information and recipes for those interested in managing Type 2 Diabetes through dietary choices. It is important to recognize that the authors and the publisher are not healthcare professionals. The suggestions and recipes contained within this book are not meant to replace professional medical advice, diagnoses, or treatments. Should you have any healthcare-related questions or concerns, particularly relating to Type 2 Diabetes management, we strongly advise consulting with your doctor or a qualified healthcare provider.

The culinary experiences, and recommendations shared in this book stem from extensive research and the personal journey of exploring dietary approaches to Type 2 Diabetes management. These narratives and suggestions are intended for educational and motivational purposes only, aiming to enhance understanding and inspire positive lifestyle changes, not to serve as direct medical or nutritional prescriptions.

The author(s) and publisher expressly disclaim any liability for any adverse effects arising directly or indirectly from the use and application of the information contained in this cookbook. Moreover, given the specificity and medical relevance of the content, certain topics and dietary advice may not be suitable for all readers. It is advisable for caregivers and adults to review the content before sharing with minors or individuals with particular sensitivities or health concerns.

In cases of medical emergencies or for immediate assistance with health issues, please reach out to a trusted healthcare professional or dial the emergency services number available in your locality.

The Entire Type 2 Diabetes Cookbook Series

Dive into a culinary revolution with the ***"Type 2 Diabetes Cookbook Series: Beginner's Quick & Easy Recipes for Delicious Diabetes Diets – 300 Health-Boosting Savory Meals for Diabetic Wellness in 30 Minutes or Less."***

Spread across six essential volumes – Breakfast, Lunch, Dinner, Desserts, Snacks, and Sauces, Dips, & Dressings – this series is your passport to a world where managing Type 2 Diabetes meets delicious innovation.

Each book is a treasure trove of hundreds of recipes, marrying the precision of nutritional science with the flair of culinary art. Designed for those on a diabetic diet, these recipes promise to transform your meals from bland to blissful without sacrificing flavor or health. Every dish, from energizing breakfasts to indulgent desserts, comes alive through vivid, full-color photographs, accompanied by foolproof instructions, cooking times, detailed ingredient lists, serving suggestions, and handy conversion charts.

But the journey doesn't end with tantalizing meals. These cookbooks are gateways to mastering diabetes management, offering insights into blood sugar balance, insulin functionality, and the art of carb counting. They stand as pillars of empowerment and knowledge, guiding you through the culinary and health aspects of diabetes with ease and enjoyment.

Embrace these cookbooks as more than mere collections of recipes; see them as companions in your journey toward diabetic wellness, bringing confidence, pleasure, and a burst of flavors into your daily life. Step into a world where managing diabetes is synonymous with culinary discovery and dietary joy. Welcome to your new kitchen adventure!

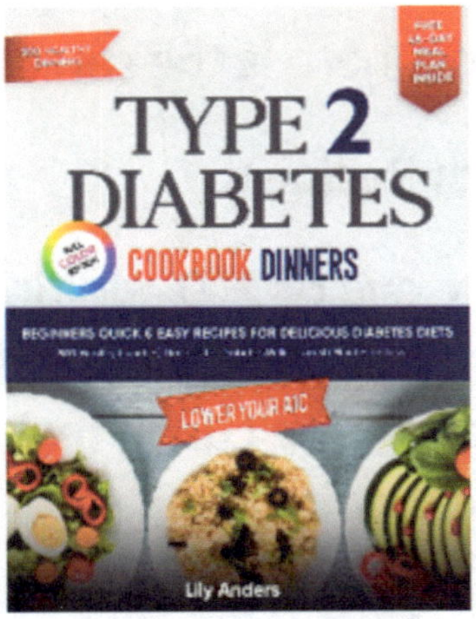
FREE 45-DAY MEAL PLAN INSIDE
TYPE 2 DIABETES
FULL COLOR EDITION
COOKBOOK DINNERS
BEGINNERS QUICK & EASY RECIPES FOR DELICIOUS DIABETES DIETS
LOWER YOUR A1C
Lily Anders

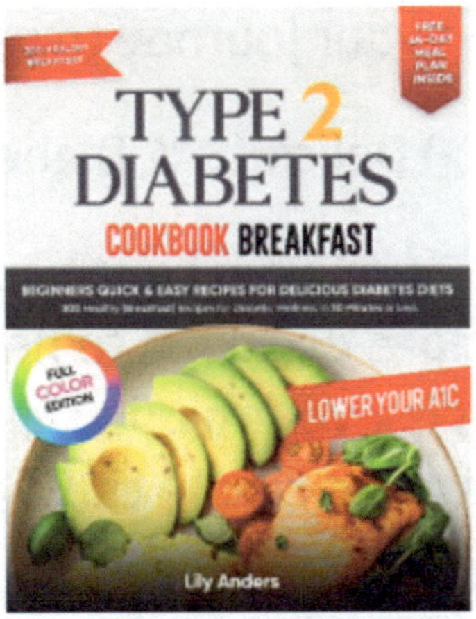
TYPE 2 DIABETES
COOKBOOK BREAKFAST
BEGINNERS QUICK & EASY RECIPES FOR DELICIOUS DIABETES DIETS
FULL COLOR EDITION
LOWER YOUR A1C
Lily Anders

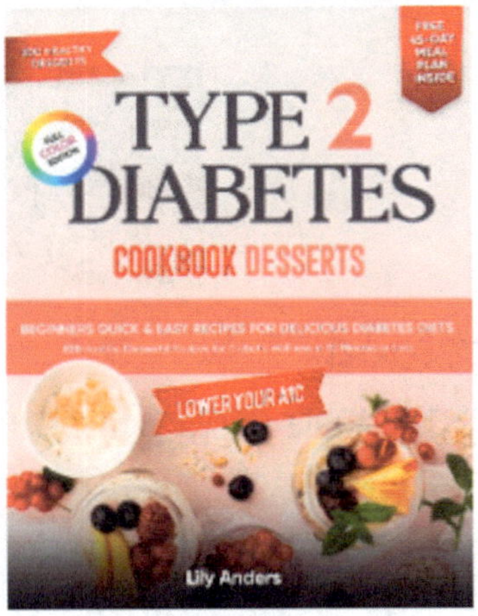
FREE 45-DAY MEAL PLAN INSIDE
TYPE 2 DIABETES
COOKBOOK DESSERTS
BEGINNERS QUICK & EASY RECIPES FOR DELICIOUS DIABETES DIETS
LOWER YOUR A1C
Lily Anders

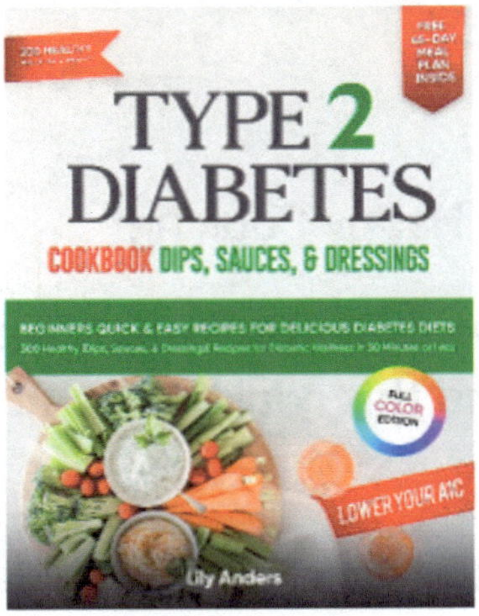
TYPE 2 DIABETES
COOKBOOK DIPS, SAUCES, & DRESSINGS
BEGINNERS QUICK & EASY RECIPES FOR DELICIOUS DIABETES DIETS
FULL COLOR EDITION
LOWER YOUR A1C
Lily Anders

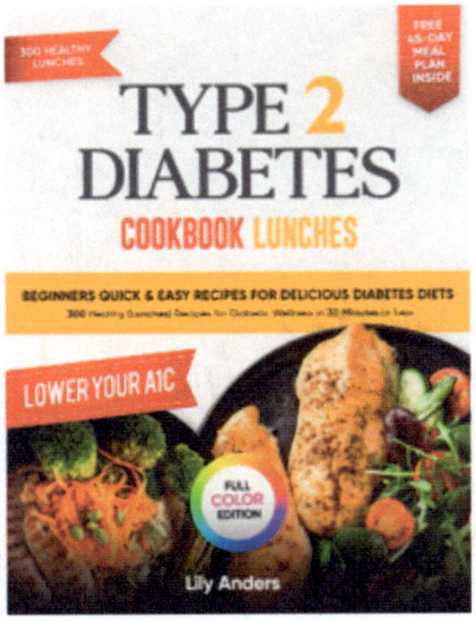
300 HEALTHY LUNCHES
FREE 45-DAY MEAL PLAN INSIDE
TYPE 2 DIABETES
COOKBOOK LUNCHES
BEGINNERS QUICK & EASY RECIPES FOR DELICIOUS DIABETES DIETS
LOWER YOUR A1C
FULL COLOR EDITION
Lily Anders

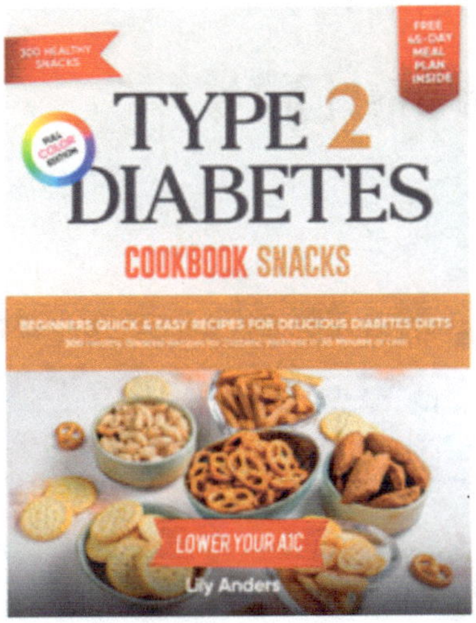
300 HEALTHY SNACKS
FREE 45-DAY MEAL PLAN INSIDE
TYPE 2 DIABETES
COOKBOOK SNACKS
BEGINNERS QUICK & EASY RECIPES FOR DELICIOUS DIABETES DIETS
LOWER YOUR A1C
Lily Anders

Here's My Promise to You!

To jumpstart your journey toward healthier eating, here is the remaining

Listing of 200 Delicious & Diabetes-Friendly Lunch Recipes!

That's right—you now have access to a treasure trove of 200 additional diabetic recipes designed to help you enjoy flavorful, balanced meals while managing your blood sugar with confidence. These Lunch recipes will inspire you to create satisfying, nutritious meals with ease.

☞ CLICK THE LINK OR SCAN THE QR CODE TO DOWNLOAD YOUR FREE RECIPE COLLECTION!

Enjoy, and Happy Cooking!

The journey to better health starts with the right food choices, and this cookbook and it is here to support you every step of the way.

Thank you for trusting this guide, and here's to a flavorful, balanced, and empowered approach to managing Type 2 Diabetes!

You've got this! ☐☐✨

<<Click here to access your 45 day meal plan>>
https://acrobat.adobe.com/id/urn:aaid:sc:VA6C2:448a7fa7-ffcd-4919-9d29-1c8e6bee62e9

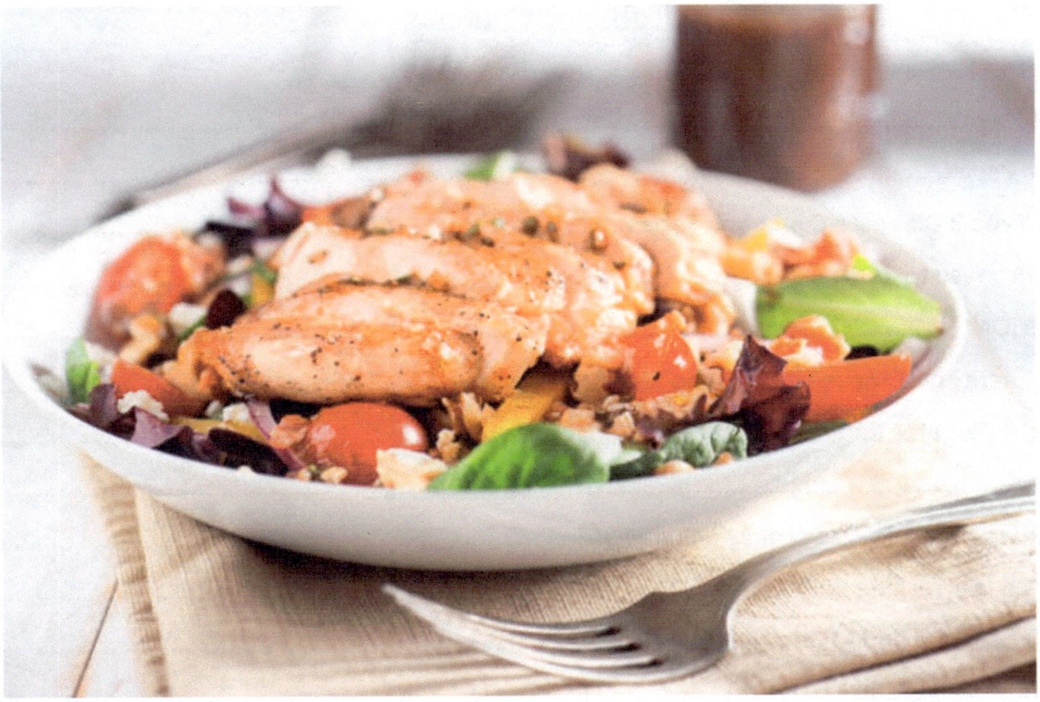

1. Grilled Chicken Salad with Balsamic Vinaigrette

Prep.Time:	**Cook Time:**	**Serving:**	**Beverage pairing:**
15 min	15 min	2	Iced Tea

Ingredients:

- 2 boneless, skinless chicken breasts
- 6 cups mixed salad greens
- 1 cup cherry tomatoes, halved
- 1/2 cup cucumber, sliced
- 1/4 cup red onion, thinly sliced
- 2 tablespoons balsamic vinegar
- 1 tablespoon olive oil
- Salt and pepper to taste

Preparation:

1. Preheat grill to medium-high heat.
2. Season chicken breasts with salt and pepper.
3. Grill chicken for 6-8 minutes per side or until cooked through.
4. Let the chicken rest for a few minutes, then slice thinly.
5. In a small bowl, whisk together balsamic vinegar, olive oil, salt, and pepper to make the vinaigrette.
6. In a large bowl, toss salad greens, cherry tomatoes, cucumber, and red onion with the vinaigrette.
7. Divide the salad onto plates and top with grilled chicken slices.

Nutrition Facts (per serving):

- Calories: 300
- Carbohydrates: 12g
- Protein: 30g
- Fat: 14g

Table of Contents

Copyright Page ... 2

Disclaimer Page ... 3

The Entire Type 2 Diabetes Cookbook Series ... 4

Here's My Promise to You! ... 6

INTRODUCTION ... 13

Sustaining Energy and Focus Through the Middle of the Day ... 13

The Type 2 Diabetes Cookbook: Lunch ... 13

Chapter 1 ... 14

Understanding Type 2 Diabetes at Midday ... 14

Why Lunch Is a Turning Point ... 14

Type 2 Diabetes and Midday Energy ... 14

Individual Needs Still Matter ... 14

Chapter 2 ... 16

Blood Sugar and the Afternoon Slump ... 16

How Lunch Triggers Energy Crashes ... 16

The Role of Balance in Midday Meals ... 16

Why Skipping Lunch Often Backfires ... 16

Working With the Midday Rhythm ... 17

Chapter 3 ... 18

Carbohydrates at Lunch Without Overload ... 18

Why Lunch Carbohydrates Feel Different ... 18

Hidden Carbohydrates in Midday Meals ... 18

Choosing Carbohydrates That Last ... 18

Pairing for Sustained Energy ... 18

Learning Through Experience ... 19

Chapter 4 ... 20

Smart Lunch Shopping ... 20

Shopping With the Workday in Mind ... 20

Navigating Packaged Lunch Foods ... 20

Building a Reliable Lunch List ... 20

Planning for Variety Without Overwhelm ... 20

Making Lunch Shopping Sustainable 21

Chapter 5 22

Prep Strategies for Busy Days 22

Preparing Ahead Without Overcomplicating 22

Building Mix-and-Match Meals 22

Using Leftovers Intentionally 22

Quick Solutions for Unpredictable Days 22

Creating a Lunch Routine That Works 23

Chapter 6 24

Portion Awareness for Sustained Energy 24

Why Lunch Portions Matter 24

Recognizing Balanced Lunch Portions 24

Common Portion Challenges at Lunch 24

Adjusting Portions Based on Your Day 24

Building Long-Term Confidence 25

Putting Midday Balance Into Practice 26

1. Grilled Chicken Salad with Balsamic Vinaigrette 27
2. Quinoa and Black Bean Bowl with Avocado 28
3. Turkey and Veggie Wrap with Whole Grain Tortilla 29
4. Mediterranean Chickpea Salad 30
5. Lemon Herb Baked Chicken with Roasted Vegetables 31
6. Salmon and Quinoa Patties with Dill Sauce 32
7. Caprese Avocado Toast with Mixed Greens 33
8. Lentil and Vegetable Soup with Spinach 34
9. Greek Yogurt Chicken Caesar Wrap 35
10. Shrimp and Broccoli Stir-Fry with Brown Rice 36
11. Chickpea and Spinach Stuffed Sweet Potatoes 37
12. Turkey and Avocado Quinoa Salad 38
13. Baked Cod with Lemon and Herbs 39
14. Veggie-loaded Quinoa and Lentil Stew 40
15. Chicken and Vegetable Skewers with Tzatziki Sauce 41
16. Zucchini Noodles with Pesto and Cherry Tomatoes 42
17. Turkey Chili with Black Beans and Tomatoes 43

18. Spinach and Feta Stuffed Bell Peppers 44
19. Asian-style Salmon Salad with Sesame Ginger Dressing..45
20. Cauliflower Rice and Chicken Burrito Bowl 46
21. Beef and Vegetable Lettuce Wraps 47
22. Grilled Eggplant and Hummus Sandwich..48
23. Quinoa and Kale Salad with Cranberries and Walnuts 49
24. Chicken and Vegetable Kebabs with Quinoa 50
25. Lentil and Mushroom Stuffed Bell Peppers 51
26. Turkey and Spinach Quesadilla with Whole Wheat Toast 52
27. Lemon Garlic Shrimp and Broccoli Bowl 53
28. Greek Chickpea and Cucumber Salad 54
29. Baked Chicken Breast with Tomato Basil Relish 55
30. Mediterranean Tuna Salad Lettuce Wraps 56
31. Vegetable and Tofu Stir-Fry with Brown Rice 57
32. Spaghetti Squash Primavera with Grilled Chicken..58
33. Turkey and Quinoa Stuffed Bell Peppers 59
34. Avocado and Chickpea Wrap with Hummus 60
35. Baked Salmon with Dijon Mustard Glaze 61
36. Tomato Basil Lentil Soup 62
37. Chicken and Vegetable Lettuce Wraps 63
38. Cauliflower and Chickpea Curry with Brown Rice..64
39. Spinach and Mushroom Quiche with Almond Flour Crust 65
40. Quinoa and Black Bean Stuffed Avocado Boats..66
41. Lemon Herb Grilled Turkey Burgers..67
42. Shrimp and Avocado Salad with Lime Vinaigrette..68
43. Greek Yogurt Chicken Pita Pocket 69
44. Quinoa and Vegetable Stir-Fry..70
45. Turkey and Cranberry Quinoa Bowl..71
46. Baked Cod with Mediterranean Salsa..72
47. Caprese Zoodle Salad with Grilled Chicken 73
48. Lentil and Vegetable Curry with Cauliflower Rice..74
49. Chicken and Black Bean Pita Bread..75
50. Spinach and Feta Turkey Burgers 76

51. Quinoa and Chickpea Salad with Lemon Tahini Dressing 80
52. Salmon and Asparagus Foil Packets 81
53. Roasted Vegetable and Hummus Wrap 82
54. Turkey and Quinoa Stuffed Acorn Squash 83
55. Chickpea and Spinach Curry with Basmati Rice 84
56. Greek Chicken and Orzo Salad 85
57. Broccoli and Cheddar Stuffed Sweet Potatoes 86
58. Turkey and Avocado Lettuce Wraps 87
59. Cauliflower Rice and Black Bean Bowl 88
60. Lemon Garlic Shrimp Pasta with Zucchini Noodles 89
61. Chicken and Vegetable Quinoa Bowl 90
62. Mediterranean Tofu Salad 91
63. Shrimp and Avocado Quinoa Bowl 92
64. Turkey and Vegetable Skillet with Quinoa 93
65. Caprese Chicken and Zucchini Noodle Bowl 94
66. Lentil and Mushroom Burgers 95
67. Grilled Lemon Herb Chicken Salad 96
68. Asian-inspired Salmon and Broccoli Bowl 97
69. Chickpea and Kale Caesar Salad 98
70. Turkey and Spinach Stuffed Mushrooms 99
71. Quinoa and Black Bean Veggie Burger 100
72. Chicken and Vegetable Stir-Fry with Cauliflower Rice 101
73. Mediterranean Chickpea and Quinoa Bowl 102
74. Turkey and Avocado Caesar Wrap 103
75. Zucchini and Tomato Frittata with Feta 104
76. Lentil and Vegetable Stuffed Pita 105
77. Salmon and Avocado Quinoa Salad 106
78. Spinach and Feta Turkey Meatballs with Greek Yogurt Sauce 107
79. Greek Chickpea and Quinoa Wrap 108
80. Teriyaki Turkey and Vegetable Skewers 109
81. Turkey and Broccoli Cauliflower Fried Rice 110
82. Caprese Chicken and Spinach Salad 111
83. Quinoa and Black Bean Enchilada Bake 112

84. Greek Yogurt Chicken and Cucumber Wrap 113
85. Squash Boat with Tomato Basil Sauce 114
86. Lentil and Vegetable Stew with Sweet Potatoes 115
87. Turkey and Cranberry Spinach Salad 116
88. Shrimp and Avocado Zoodle Bowl 117
89. Chickpea and Vegetable Curry with Quinoa 118
90. Turkey and Pesto Zucchini Noodle Bowl....................119
91. Mediterranean Tuna and White Bean Salad....................120
92. Chicken and Vegetable Burrito 121
93. Quinoa and Black Bean Stuffed Bell Pepper 122
94. Grilled Lemon Herb Turkey Skewers....................123
95. Caprese Eggplant and Spinach Stack 124
96. Baked Salmon with Cucumber Dill Salad 125
97. Lentil and Vegetable Curry Stuffed Acorn Squash....................126
98. Turkey and Avocado Caesar Salad 127
99. Quinoa and Black Bean Tacos with Greek Yogurt Sauce 128
100. Chicken and Broccoli Cauliflower Rice Casserole 129

INTRODUCTION

Sustaining Energy and Focus Through the Middle of the Day

For many people managing Type 2 Diabetes, lunch is the most overlooked meal of the day. Mornings may begin with good intentions, but by midday, schedules tighten, energy dips, and decisions are rushed. Lunch often becomes something eaten quickly, postponed, or improvised.

Yet lunch plays a critical role in how the rest of the day unfolds.

A well-balanced lunch supports steady blood sugar levels, sustained energy, and mental clarity through the afternoon. An unbalanced or skipped lunch often leads to fatigue, cravings, irritability, or overeating later in the day. For individuals with Type 2 Diabetes, these patterns can make management feel harder than it needs to be.

This book was written for that moment in the day.

The Type 2 Diabetes Cookbook: Lunch is designed to bring structure and confidence to midday meals. It focuses on practical, diabetes-conscious lunches that fit into real workdays, errands, and busy schedules. These meals are intended to support blood sugar balance without requiring excessive preparation or complicated planning.

Lunch is unique because it must fuel activity rather than rest. Unlike dinner, which prepares the body for winding down, lunch is meant to sustain focus, productivity, and steady energy. This requires a thoughtful balance of protein, fiber, and controlled carbohydrates that nourish without slowing you down.

The good news is that supportive lunches do not need to be boring, repetitive, or time-consuming.

In this book, you will find lunch recipes that are satisfying without being heavy and flexible enough to adapt to different routines. Meals are created to be prepared quickly, packed easily, and enjoyed wherever your day takes you.

This cookbook is not about rigid meal timing or perfect choices. It is about building dependable lunch habits that work consistently, even on busy days. Whether you eat lunch at home, at work, or on the go, these recipes are meant to support you.

You will not be asked to overthink every ingredient or track every bite. Instead, you will learn patterns that help lunch become a stabilizing point in your day rather than a source of stress.

When lunch works, afternoons feel smoother, cravings feel quieter, and evenings become easier to manage.

Welcome to a clearer, more confident approach to midday meals with Type 2 Diabetes.

Chapter 1

Understanding Type 2 Diabetes at Midday

By lunchtime, your body has already responded to the foods and activities of the morning. Blood sugar levels have risen and fallen, energy has been spent, and insulin has been at work. For individuals managing Type 2 Diabetes, the midday period is often where imbalances begin to show.

Type 2 Diabetes affects how the body uses insulin, the hormone responsible for moving glucose from the bloodstream into the cells. When insulin does not work efficiently, glucose remains in the blood longer than it should, leading to elevated blood sugar levels. This process continues throughout the day, influenced by meals, movement, stress, and timing.

Lunch plays a critical role in this ongoing process.

Why Lunch Is a Turning Point

Unlike breakfast, which follows an overnight fast, lunch arrives after the body has already been active. Physical movement, mental effort, and stress all increase energy demands. If lunch does not provide balanced fuel, the body may respond with fatigue, irritability, or difficulty concentrating during the afternoon.

A lunch that is high in refined carbohydrates and low in protein or fiber may cause blood sugar levels to rise quickly, followed by a noticeable drop. This pattern often contributes to what many people describe as the afternoon slump.

When lunch is balanced, blood sugar responses are steadier, energy lasts longer, and cravings later in the day are reduced.

Type 2 Diabetes and Midday Energy

Managing Type 2 Diabetes is not only about blood sugar numbers. It is also about how you feel and function throughout the day. Lunch has a direct influence on productivity, focus, and mood.

Meals that are too light may leave you hungry soon after eating. Meals that are too heavy may cause sluggishness. Finding the middle ground is essential.

Balanced lunches provide enough nourishment to sustain energy without overwhelming the digestive system. This balance supports better blood sugar control and a more consistent afternoon rhythm.

Individual Needs Still Matter

Just as with breakfast, there is no single perfect lunch for everyone. Activity level, work schedule, stress, and personal food preferences all play a role in how meals are processed.

This book does not promote rigid rules. Instead, it offers patterns that work for most people managing Type 2 Diabetes. These patterns can be adjusted as needed to fit your lifestyle.

The goal is not perfection. The goal is consistency.

In the next chapter, we will explore how blood sugar behaves during the afternoon hours and why certain lunch combinations help prevent energy crashes and cravings.

Chapter 2

Blood Sugar and the Afternoon Slump

For many people managing Type 2 Diabetes, the afternoon hours present a familiar challenge. Energy fades, focus declines, and cravings begin to surface. This pattern is often blamed on a long day or lack of sleep, but in many cases, lunch choices play a significant role.

After eating lunch, blood sugar levels naturally rise as food is digested and glucose enters the bloodstream. Insulin is released to help move this glucose into the cells. When this process happens gradually, energy remains steady. When it happens too quickly, the result is often a sharp rise followed by an equally sharp drop.

This rise and fall is commonly experienced as the afternoon slump.

How Lunch Triggers Energy Crashes

Meals that rely heavily on refined carbohydrates, such as white bread, pasta, or sugary sauces, are digested rapidly. When these foods are not balanced with protein, fiber, or healthy fats, glucose enters the bloodstream quickly. Blood sugar levels spike, insulin responds aggressively, and energy soon dips.

This cycle may leave you feeling tired, unfocused, or hungry within a short period of time. For individuals with Type 2 Diabetes, these fluctuations can feel more intense and harder to manage.

The issue is not eating lunch. The issue is how lunch is composed.

The Role of Balance in Midday Meals

Balanced lunches support steady digestion and more predictable blood sugar responses. Protein slows the release of glucose, fiber adds structure to digestion, and healthy fats provide lasting satisfaction.

When these elements are present, blood sugar rises more gently and energy lasts longer. This steadiness reduces cravings and helps prevent overeating later in the day.

Balanced lunches also support mental clarity. When blood sugar remains stable, focus and decision-making tend to improve, making the afternoon more manageable.

Why Skipping Lunch Often Backfires

Some individuals choose to skip lunch in an effort to avoid blood sugar fluctuations. While this may seem helpful in the short term, it often creates additional challenges.

Skipping lunch can lead to intense hunger later in the day, increasing the likelihood of overeating at dinner or snacking impulsively. It may also cause blood sugar levels to fluctuate as the body compensates for prolonged periods without food.

Eating a balanced lunch provides structure and helps maintain consistent energy throughout the afternoon.

Working With the Midday Rhythm

The body follows natural daily rhythms that influence digestion and energy use. Lunch plays an important role in maintaining these rhythms.

When lunch is predictable and balanced, the body responds with improved regulation. Energy feels steadier, focus improves, and the transition into the evening becomes smoother.

This book emphasizes lunches that support sustained energy rather than quick fullness. Meals are designed to be satisfying without being heavy and practical without being complicated.

In the next chapter, we will explore carbohydrates at lunch, how to approach them without overload, and how portion awareness can help maintain balance through the afternoon.

Chapter 3

Carbohydrates at Lunch Without Overload

Carbohydrates are often the most challenging part of lunch for individuals managing Type 2 Diabetes. Sandwiches, wraps, pasta dishes, and sides are common at midday, making it easy for carbohydrate intake to increase without notice.

The goal at lunch is not to eliminate carbohydrates. It is to use them intentionally, in ways that support steady energy and blood sugar balance through the afternoon.

Why Lunch Carbohydrates Feel Different

Unlike breakfast, lunch occurs after the body has already been active for several hours. Energy demands are higher, and hunger may be stronger. This can make it tempting to rely on quick, carbohydrate-heavy meals for immediate satisfaction.

However, carbohydrates consumed in large amounts or without balance can overwhelm the body's ability to regulate blood sugar. This often results in energy dips, cravings, and difficulty concentrating later in the day.

Understanding how to manage carbohydrates at lunch helps prevent these outcomes.

Hidden Carbohydrates in Midday Meals

Many lunch foods contain more carbohydrates than expected. Breads, tortillas, sauces, dressings, and side items can quietly add up.

Even meals that appear healthy may be carbohydrate-heavy when portions are large or ingredients are not balanced. Being aware of these hidden sources helps you make informed choices without feeling restricted.

This awareness is not about counting every gram. It is about recognizing patterns that affect how you feel after eating.

Choosing Carbohydrates That Last

Whole grains, legumes, vegetables, and fruits provide carbohydrates that digest more slowly due to their fiber content. These foods support more stable blood sugar responses when paired with protein and healthy fats.

For example, a lunch built around vegetables, lean protein, and a moderate portion of whole grains provides more lasting energy than one centered on refined starches alone.

The quality of carbohydrates matters as much as the quantity.

Pairing for Sustained Energy

Pairing carbohydrates with protein and fat is especially important at lunch. Protein supports muscle and tissue needs during the day, while healthy fats contribute to satiety and slower digestion.

A balanced lunch might include a protein-rich main item, fiber-rich vegetables, and a moderate carbohydrate portion. This combination helps prevent rapid blood sugar changes and keeps energy steady into the afternoon.

These pairings allow carbohydrates to be included without overload.

Learning Through Experience

Each person responds differently to carbohydrates in lunch. Activity level, stress, and individual metabolism all influence how meals are processed.

This book encourages you to observe your responses rather than follow rigid rules. If a meal leaves you energized and satisfied, it is likely well-balanced. If it leads to fatigue or cravings, small adjustments can improve the outcome.

In the next chapter, we will focus on smart lunch shopping, helping you choose ingredients that make balanced midday meals easier to prepare and enjoy.

Chapter 4

Smart Lunch Shopping

Lunch shopping presents unique challenges for individuals managing Type 2 Diabetes. Midday meals are often influenced by time constraints, work schedules, and convenience, making it easy to rely on processed or last-minute options. Shopping with intention helps reduce these pressures and makes balanced lunches easier to achieve.

Smart lunch shopping is not about perfection. It is about choosing ingredients that support steady energy and blood sugar balance while fitting into real-life routines.

Shopping With the Workday in Mind

Many lunches are eaten away from home, at work, in the car, or between commitments. When shopping, it is helpful to prioritize foods that travel well and require minimal preparation.

Lean proteins such as cooked chicken, turkey, tuna, eggs, and legumes form the backbone of balanced lunches. These items can be used in salads, wraps, bowls, or eaten on their own. Having protein readily available makes it easier to build satisfying meals without relying on carbohydrate-heavy options.

Pre-cut vegetables, salad greens, and frozen vegetables save time and reduce barriers to healthier choices. These ingredients can be combined quickly with proteins to create complete meals.

Navigating Packaged Lunch Foods

Packaged foods are common at lunch, but not all options support blood sugar stability. Many packaged meals, soups, and snack-style lunches contain refined carbohydrates, added sugars, and high sodium levels.

When choosing packaged items, focus on those with simple ingredient lists and a balance of protein and fiber. Avoid products that rely heavily on white flour, sugar, or sugary sauces.

Dressings and condiments deserve special attention. These items often contain hidden sugars and can significantly increase carbohydrate intake. Choosing simple dressings or making your own allows for greater control.

Building a Reliable Lunch List

Creating a consistent list of lunch-friendly foods reduces decision fatigue and impulse purchases. This list might include proteins, vegetables, whole grains, and healthy fats that you enjoy and can use in multiple combinations.

Shopping with a plan helps prevent the common midday question of what to eat. When the refrigerator and pantry are stocked with reliable options, balanced lunches become the default rather than the exception.

Planning for Variety Without Overwhelm

Variety is important, but too many choices can be overwhelming. Selecting a small rotation of lunch staples provides balance without complexity.

For example, a few protein options, several vegetables, and one or two carbohydrate sources can be mixed and matched throughout the week. This approach supports consistency while still allowing flexibility.

Making Lunch Shopping Sustainable

Effective lunch shopping supports long-term success. As you become familiar with dependable ingredients, shopping becomes quicker and more intuitive.

Over time, your environment begins to work in your favor. Balanced lunches feel easier to prepare, and midday energy becomes more predictable.

In the next chapter, we will explore simple preparation strategies that make it easier to assemble lunches during busy days, reducing stress and supporting consistency.

Chapter 5

Prep Strategies for Busy Days

Busy days often make lunch feel like an afterthought. Meetings, errands, deadlines, and unexpected interruptions can quickly push balanced meals aside. For individuals managing Type 2 Diabetes, this pattern can lead to skipped meals, rushed choices, or reliance on convenience foods that do not support blood sugar stability.

Simple preparation strategies help prevent these challenges and make consistent lunches easier to maintain.

Preparing Ahead Without Overcomplicating

Meal preparation does not need to be time-consuming or rigid. Even small steps taken in advance can significantly reduce stress during the day.

Cooking proteins ahead of time, such as chicken, fish, beans, or tofu, provides a foundation for quick meals. These proteins can be paired with vegetables, grains, or salads in different combinations throughout the week.

Washing and chopping vegetables in advance makes assembly faster and encourages healthier choices. When ingredients are ready to use, it becomes easier to put together a balanced lunch in minutes.

Building Mix-and-Match Meals

One effective strategy for busy days is creating meals that can be assembled rather than cooked from scratch. Mix-and-match lunches allow flexibility without requiring daily planning.

A typical mix-and-match approach includes one protein, one or two vegetables, and a moderate carbohydrate source. These components can be combined in bowls, wraps, or salads, depending on preference.

This method reduces decision fatigue while still allowing variety.

Using Leftovers Intentionally

Leftovers can be a valuable lunch resource when planned intentionally. Cooking slightly larger portions at dinner provides ready-made lunches for the next day.

The key is balance. Leftover meals should include protein, vegetables, and portions of controlled carbohydrates. When leftovers are already balanced, they require little adjustment for lunch.

Storing leftovers in individual containers makes them easier to grab and take along.

Quick Solutions for Unpredictable Days

Not every day allows for planned meals. Keeping a few reliable backup options on hand helps prevent skipped lunches or impulsive choices.

Shelf-stable items such as canned tuna, nuts, seeds, and whole-grain crackers can be combined quickly. Carefully chosen frozen meals can also be a practical option when time is limited.

These backups are not a replacement for regular meals but a support for challenging days.

Creating a Lunch Routine That Works

Consistency improves blood sugar management and reduces stress. Developing a simple lunch routine helps make balanced meals feel automatic rather than effortful.

This routine does not need to look the same every day. It simply provides structure and predictability.

In the next chapter, we will focus on portion awareness at lunch, helping you eat enough to sustain energy without feeling overly full or sluggish in the afternoon.

Chapter 6

Portion Awareness for Sustained Energy

Portion size plays a critical role in how lunch affects energy, focus, and blood sugar levels. Even balanced foods can lead to discomfort or fatigue when portions are larger than the body needs, especially in the middle of the day.

Portion awareness at lunch is not about restriction. It is about finding the amount that supports steady energy without causing heaviness or sluggishness.

Why Lunch Portions Matter

After eating lunch, the body shifts energy toward digestion. When portions are too large, digestion can feel demanding, pulling energy away from mental focus and physical activity. This often results in feelings of sleepiness or reduced productivity.

For individuals managing Type 2 Diabetes, large portions of carbohydrates can also lead to sharper blood sugar rises, followed by drops that affect energy and mood.

Balanced portions help maintain a smoother blood sugar response and support consistent energy through the afternoon.

Recognizing Balanced Lunch Portions

A balanced lunch typically includes protein, vegetables, and a moderate amount of carbohydrates. Protein helps slow digestion and promotes fullness, while vegetables provide fiber that supports blood sugar stability.

Carbohydrates should be present but controlled. Portions that feel satisfying without feeling heavy are often most effective.

Visual cues can be helpful. A plate that includes a generous portion of vegetables, a solid protein source, and a smaller portion of grains or starches often provides a good balance.

Common Portion Challenges at Lunch

Lunch portions can easily increase due to distractions, eating quickly, or relying on packaged meals. Sandwiches, wraps, and bowls often contain more food than expected, especially when combined with sides.

Eating while working or multitasking can make it harder to recognize fullness. Taking a moment to pause during meals can improve portion awareness and satisfaction.

These challenges are common and manageable with practice.

Adjusting Portions Based on Your Day

Portion needs may vary depending on activity level, stress, and timing of meals. On more active days, slightly larger portions may be appropriate. On less active days, smaller portions may feel more comfortable.

Listening to your body and adjusting as needed supports flexibility without losing structure.

This approach encourages consistency rather than perfection.

Building Long-Term Confidence

As portion awareness improves, lunch becomes easier to manage. Over time, you will begin to recognize the amount of food that supports steady energy without discomfort.

The recipes in this book are designed with portion awareness in mind, helping remove much of the guesswork.

In the next section, we will transition into the lunch recipes, where these principles are put into practice through practical, satisfying meals designed for busy days.

Putting Midday Balance Into Practice

The guidance you have explored so far is meant to simplify your lunch decisions, not complicate them. Understanding how Type 2 Diabetes affects midday energy, learning to approach carbohydrates with intention, and developing realistic habits around shopping, preparation, and portion awareness all serve one goal, and that is to help you move through the afternoon with steadiness and confidence.

Now it is time to put these principles into action.

The lunch recipes that follow are designed to support sustained energy and blood sugar balance during busy days. Each recipe emphasizes practical combinations of protein, fiber, and carbohydrates, helping you feel satisfied without feeling heavy or sluggish. Meals are created to be approachable, flexible, and realistic for workdays, errands, and active schedules.

You do not need to prepare every recipe or follow them in sequence. Choose options that fit your routine and preferences. Some lunches may be eaten at home, others packed to go, and some enjoyed between commitments. All are designed with consistency and ease in mind.

As you explore the recipes, pay attention to how different meals support your focus, energy, and hunger levels throughout the afternoon. Use that awareness to guide future choices, making small adjustments as needed.

This section is not about strict rules or perfect execution. It is about building reliable lunch habits that support your health while fitting naturally into your day.

Let these recipes help carry you through the afternoon with clarity, balance, and confidence.

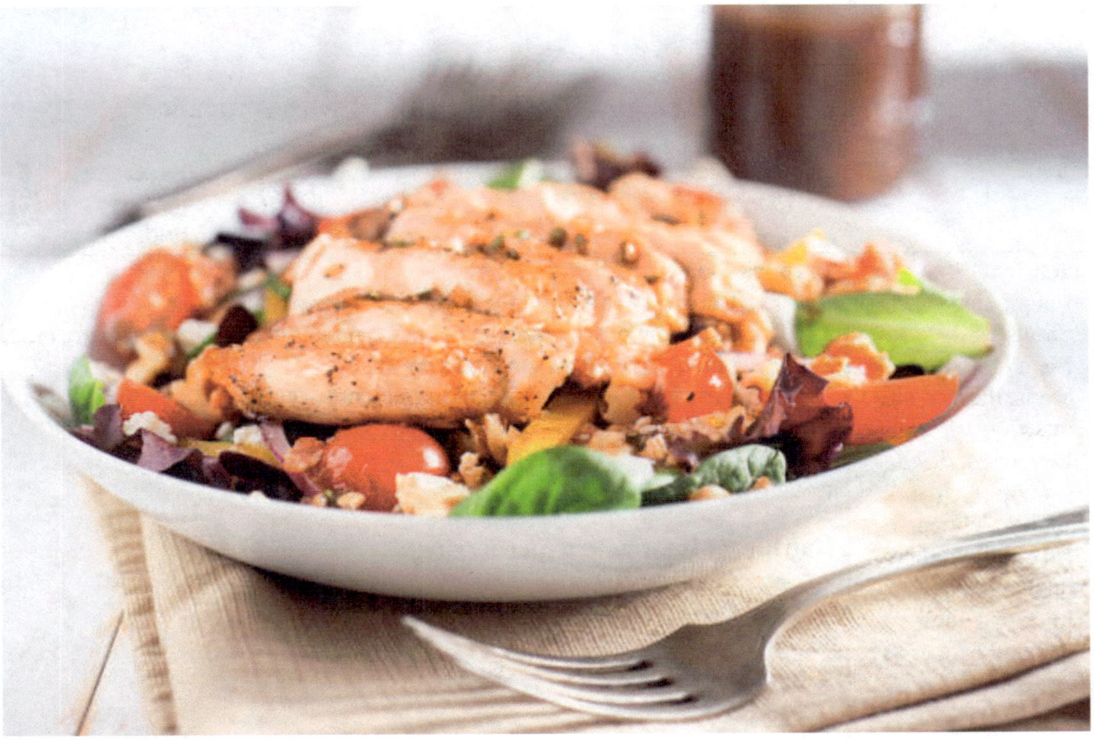

1. Grilled Chicken Salad with Balsamic Vinaigrette

Prep.Time: 15 min

Cook Time: 15 min

Serving: 2

Beverage pairing: Iced Tea

Ingredients:

- 2 boneless, skinless chicken breasts
- 6 cups mixed salad greens
- 1 cup cherry tomatoes, halved
- 1/2 cup cucumber, sliced
- 1/4 cup red onion, thinly sliced
- 2 tablespoons balsamic vinegar
- 1 tablespoon olive oil
- Salt and pepper to taste

Preparation:

1. Preheat grill to medium-high heat.
2. Season chicken breasts with salt and pepper.
3. Grill chicken for 6-8 minutes per side or until cooked through.
4. Let the chicken rest for a few minutes, then slice thinly.
5. In a small bowl, whisk together balsamic vinegar, olive oil, salt, and pepper to make the vinaigrette.
6. In a large bowl, toss salad greens, cherry tomatoes, cucumber, and red onion with the vinaigrette.
7. Divide the salad onto plates and top with grilled chicken slices.

Nutrition Facts (per serving):

- Calories: 300
- Carbohydrates: 12g
- Protein: 30g
- Fat: 14g

2. Quinoa and Black Bean Bowl with Avocado

Prep.Time: 20 min | **Cook Time:** 15 min | **Serving:** 2 | **Beverage pairing:** Herbal Tea

Ingredients:

- 1 cup quinoa, rinsed
- 1 can (15 oz) black beans, drained and rinsed
- 1 avocado, diced
- 1/4 cup fresh cilantro, chopped
- 1/4 cup red onion, finely chopped
- Juice of 1 lime
- Salt and pepper to taste

Preparation:

1. Cook quinoa according to package instructions.
2. In a large bowl, combine cooked quinoa, black beans, avocado, cilantro, red onion, lime juice, salt, and pepper.
3. Toss gently to combine all ingredients evenly.

Nutritional Information (per serving):

- Calories: 100
- Carbohydrates: 10g
- Fat: 7g
- Protein: 2g

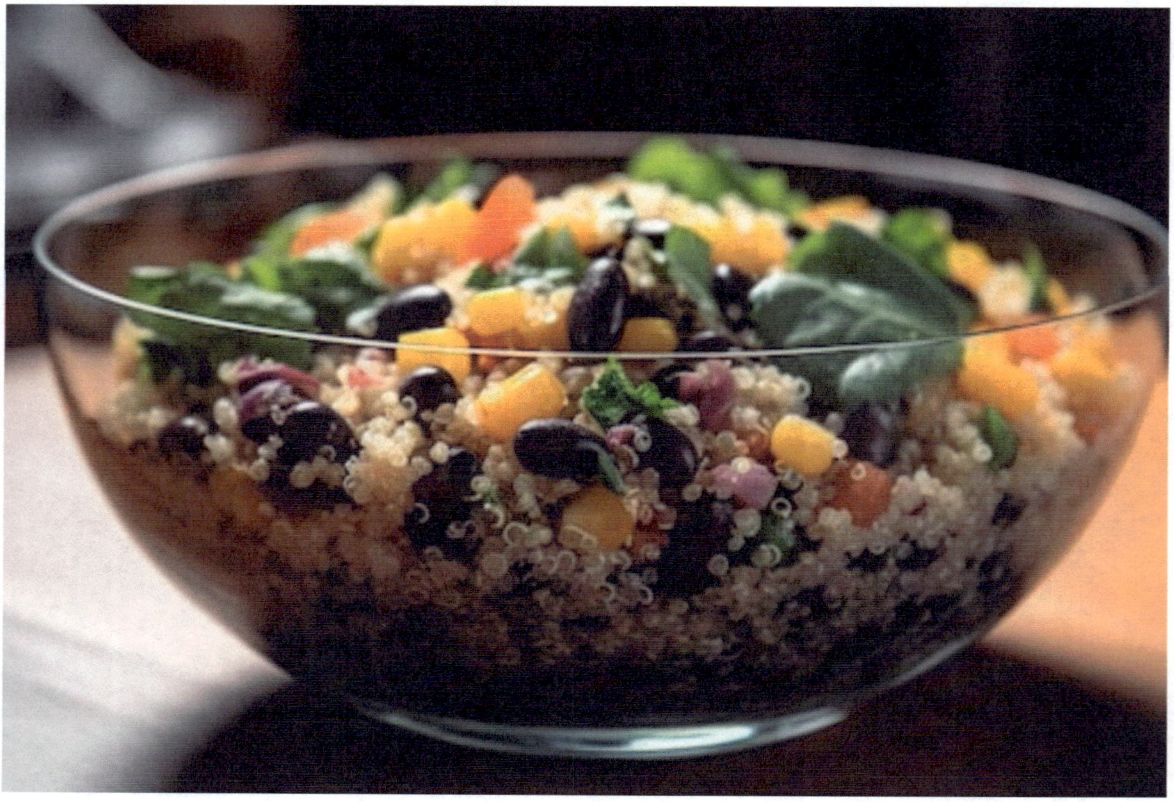

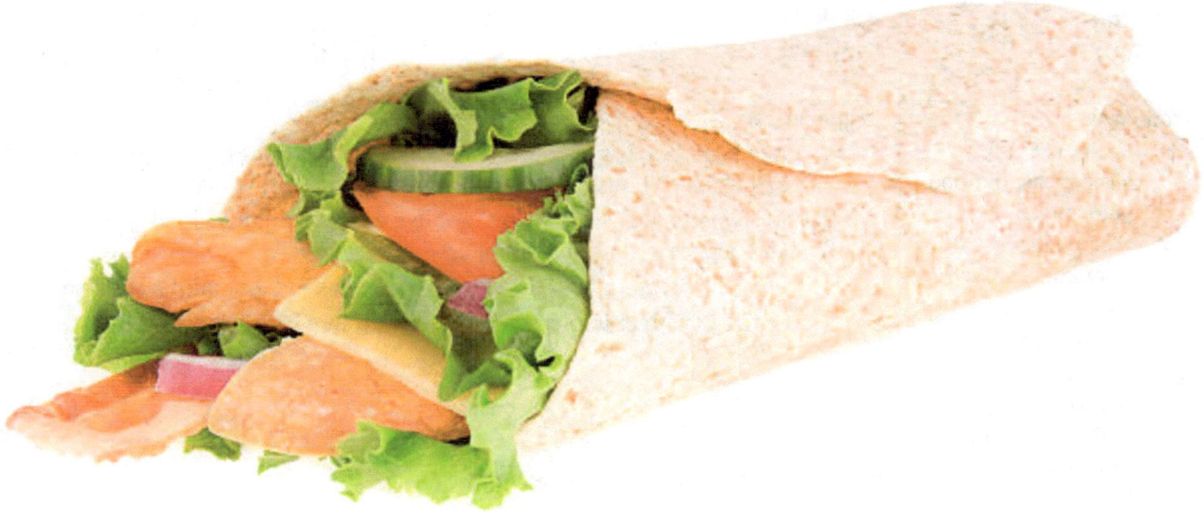

3. Turkey and Veggie Wrap with Whole Grain Tortilla

Prep.Time:	Cook Time:	Serving:	Beverage pairing:
10 min	0 min	2	HerbalTea

Ingredients:

- 2 whole grain tortillas
- 6 oz sliced turkey breast
- 1/2 cup mixed salad greens
- 1/4 cup cucumber, sliced
- 1/4 cup bell peppers, thinly sliced
- 1/4 cup shredded carrots
- 2 tablespoons hummus

Preparation:

1. Lay out the tortillas on a clean surface.
2. Spread 1 tablespoon of hummus onto each tortilla.
3. Layer sliced turkey, mixed salad greens, cucumber, bell peppers, and shredded carrots evenly on each tortilla.
4. Roll up the tortillas tightly, tucking in the sides as you go.
5. Slice each wrap in half diagonally and serve.

Nutrition Facts (per serving):

- Calories: 320
- Carbohydrates: 35g
- Protein: 22g
- Fat: 11g

4. Mediterranean Chickpea Salad

Prep.Time: 15 min

Cook Time: 0 min

Serving: 2

Beverage pairing: Lemonade

Ingredients:

- 1 can (15 oz) chickpeas, drained and rinsed
- 1 cup cherry tomatoes, halved
- 1/2 English cucumber, diced
- 1/4 cup red onion, thinly sliced
- 1/4 cup Kalamata olives, pitted and halved
- 2 tablespoons extra virgin olive oil
- 1 tablespoon lemon juice
- 1 teaspoon dried oregano
- Salt and pepper to taste
- 2 tablespoons crumbled feta cheese (optional)

Preparation:

1. In a large bowl, combine chickpeas, cherry tomatoes, cucumber, red onion, and Kalamata olives.
2. In a small bowl, whisk together olive oil, lemon juice, dried oregano, salt, and pepper to make the dressing.
3. Pour the dressing over the chickpea mixture and toss until evenly coated.
4. Sprinkle with crumbled feta cheese if desired before serving.

Nutritional Information (per serving):

- Calories: 280
- Carbohydrates: 28g
- Protein: 9g
- Fat: 15g

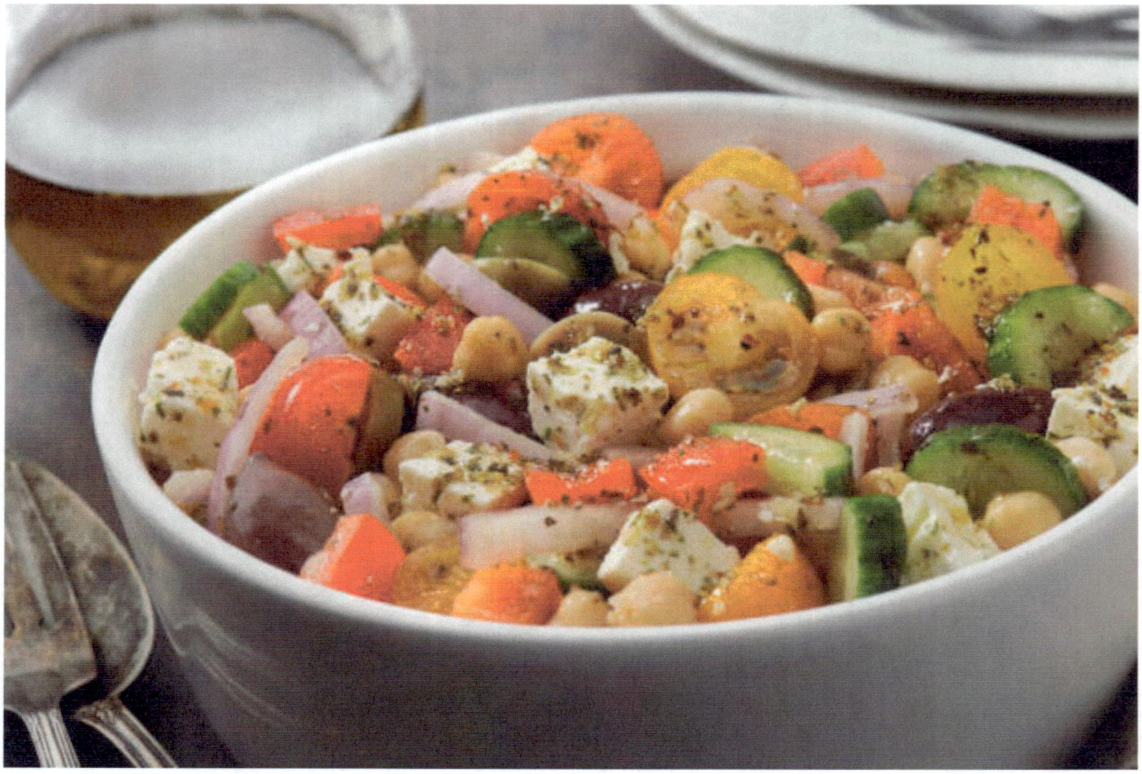

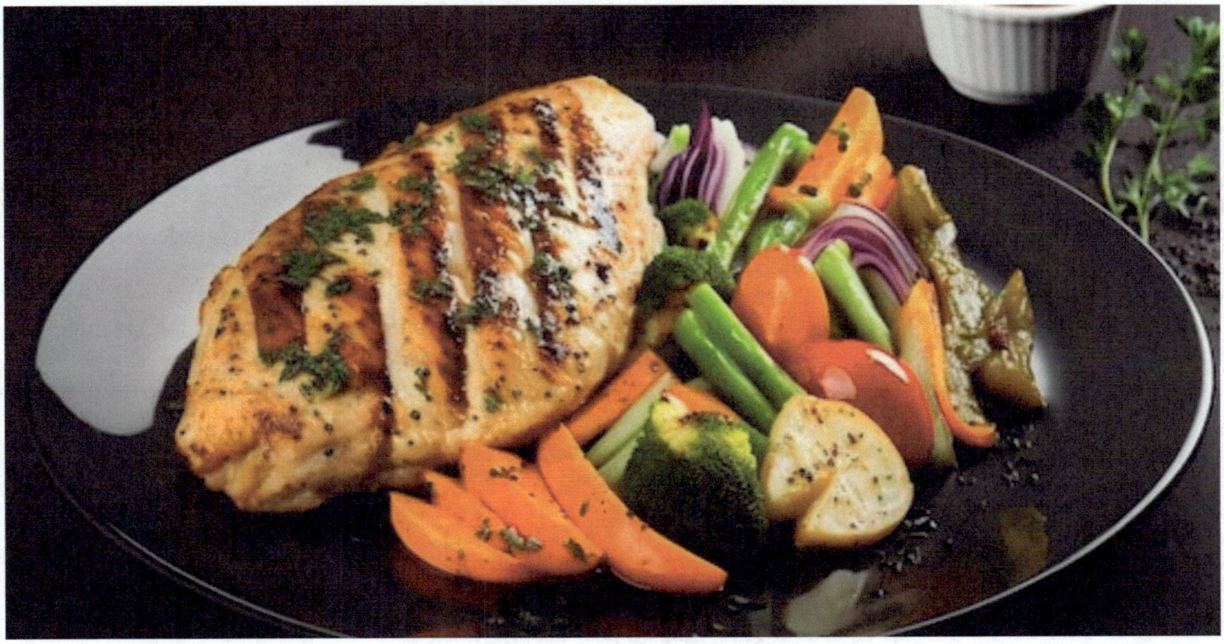

5. Lemon Herb Baked Chicken with Roasted Vegetables

Prep.Time: 15 min | **Cook Time:** 25 min | **Serving:** 2 | **Beverage pairing:** GreenlTea

Ingredients:

- 2 boneless, skinless chicken breasts (about 8 oz each)
- 2 cups mixed vegetables (such as bell peppers, zucchini, and broccoli), chopped
- 2 tablespoons olive oil
- 1 tablespoon fresh lemon juice
- 1 teaspoon dried thyme
- 1 teaspoon dried rosemary
- Salt and pepper to taste

Preparation:

1. Preheat oven to 400°F (200°C).
2. In a small bowl, whisk together olive oil, lemon juice, dried thyme, dried rosemary, salt, and pepper to make the marinade.
3. Place chicken breasts in a baking dish and pour half of the marinade over them, turning to coat evenly. Let them marinate for 10 minutes.
4. Arrange chopped vegetables around the chicken in the baking dish. Drizzle the remaining marinade over the vegetables.
5. Bake for 20-25 minutes, or until chicken is cooked through and vegetables are tender.

Nutrition Facts (per serving):

- Calories: 320
- Carbohydrates: 12g
- Protein: 35g
- Fat: 15g

6. Salmon and Quinoa Patties with Dill Sauce

Prep.Time: 20 min

Cook Time: 10 min

Serving: 2

Beverage pairing: Herbal Tea

Ingredients:

- 1 can (6 oz) salmon, drained and flaked
- 1 cup cooked quinoa
- 1/4 cup breadcrumbs
- 1 egg, beaten
- 2 tablespoons chopped fresh dill
- Salt and pepper to taste
- 1 tablespoon olive oil
- 1/4 cup plain Greek yogurt
- 1 tablespoon fresh lemon juice
- 1 tablespoon chopped fresh dill
- Salt and pepper to taste

Preparation:

1. In a large bowl, mix together salmon, cooked quinoa, breadcrumbs, beaten egg, chopped dill, salt, and pepper until well combined.
2. Form the mixture into patties.
3. Heat olive oil in a skillet over medium heat. Cook patties for 3-4 minutes per side, or until golden brown and heated through.
4. For the dill sauce, mix together Greek yogurt, lemon juice, chopped dill, salt, and pepper in a small bowl.
5. Serve salmon and quinoa patties with dill sauce on the side.

Nutritional Information (per serving):

- Calories: 300
- Carbohydrates: 20g
- Protein: 20g
- Fat: 15g

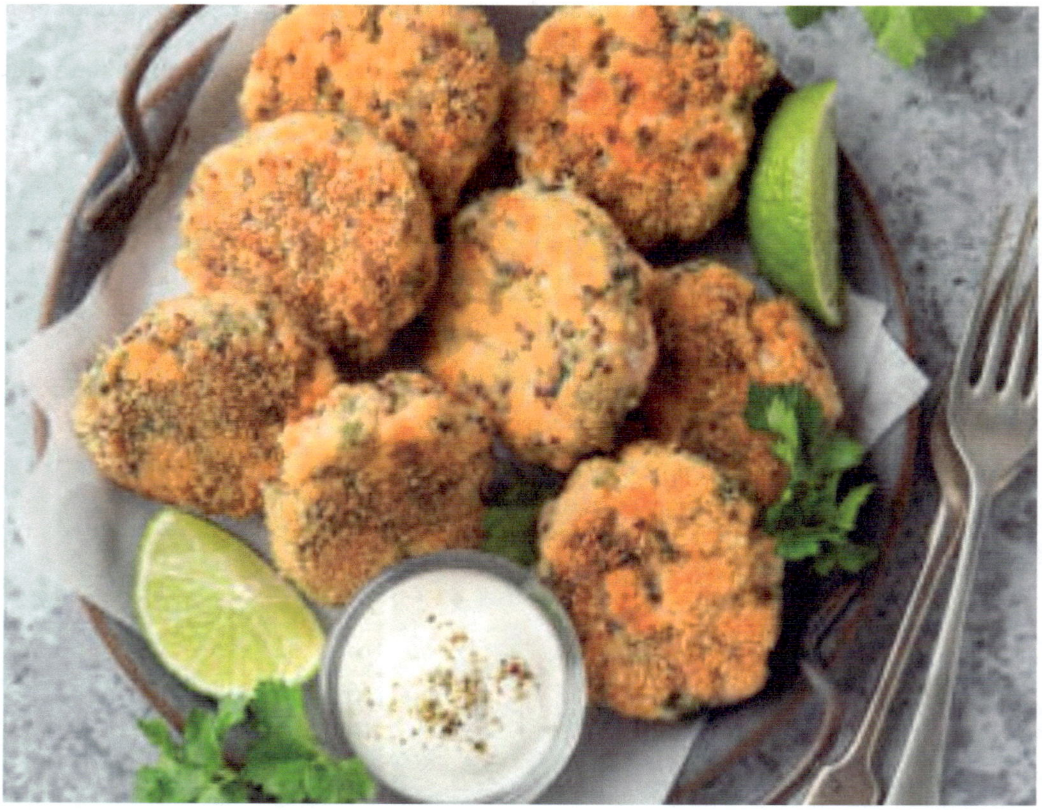

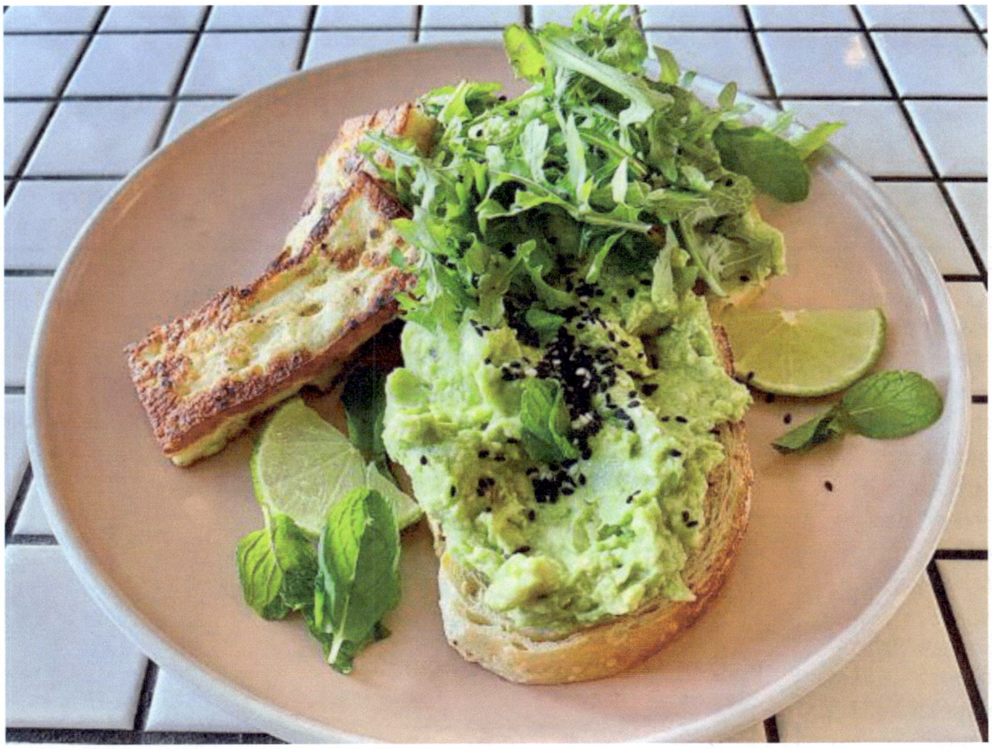

7. Caprese Avocado Toast with Mixed Greens

Prep.Time: 10 min

Cook Time: 0 min

Serving: 2

Beverage pairing: Milk

Ingredients:

- 2 slices whole grain bread, toasted
- 1 ripe avocado, mashed
- 1 large tomato, sliced
- 2 slices fresh mozzarella cheese
- 1/4 cup fresh basil leaves
- Salt and pepper to taste
- Mixed greens for serving

Preparation:

1. Spread mashed avocado evenly onto each slice of toasted bread.
2. Top with sliced tomato, fresh mozzarella cheese, and basil leaves.
3. Season with salt and pepper to taste.
4. Serve with a side of mixed greens.

Nutrition Facts (per serving):

- Calories: 350
- Carbohydrates: 25g
- Protein: 12g
- Fat: 22g

8. Lentil and Vegetable Soup with Spinach

Prep.Time: 10 min

Cook Time: 30 min

Serving: 4

Beverage pairing: Herbal Tea

Ingredients:

- 1 cup dry green lentils, rinsed and drained
- 4 cups vegetable broth
- 1 onion, diced
- 2 carrots, diced
- 2 celery stalks, diced
- 2 garlic cloves, minced
- 1 teaspoon dried thyme
- 1 teaspoon dried oregano
- 2 cups fresh spinach leaves
- Salt and pepper to taste

Preparation:

1. In a large pot, combine lentils, vegetable broth, diced onion, carrots, celery, minced garlic, dried thyme, and dried oregano.
2. Bring to a boil, then reduce heat and simmer for 20-25 minutes, or until lentils and vegetables are tender.
3. Stir in fresh spinach leaves and cook for an additional 2-3 minutes until wilted.
4. Season with salt and pepper to taste before serving.

Nutritional Information (per serving):

- Calories: 250
- Carbohydrates: 45g
- Protein: 15g
- Fat: 2g

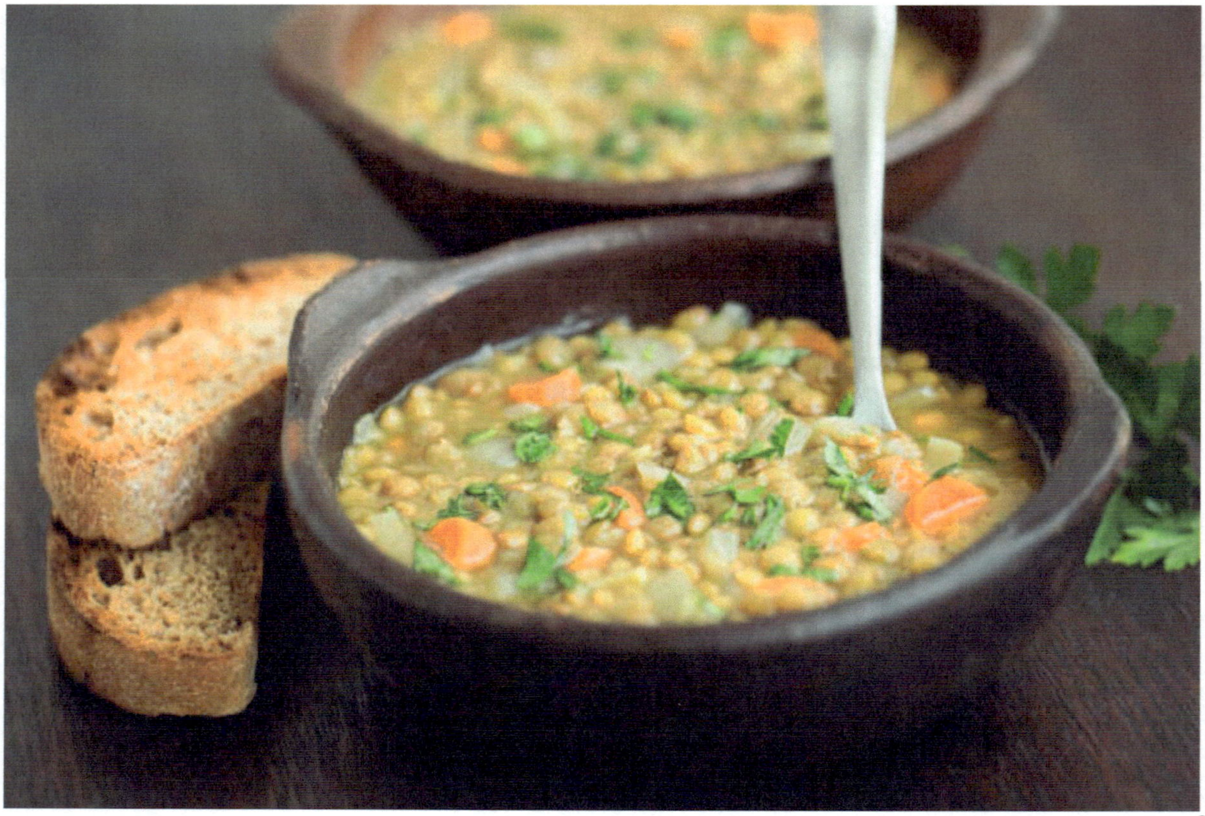

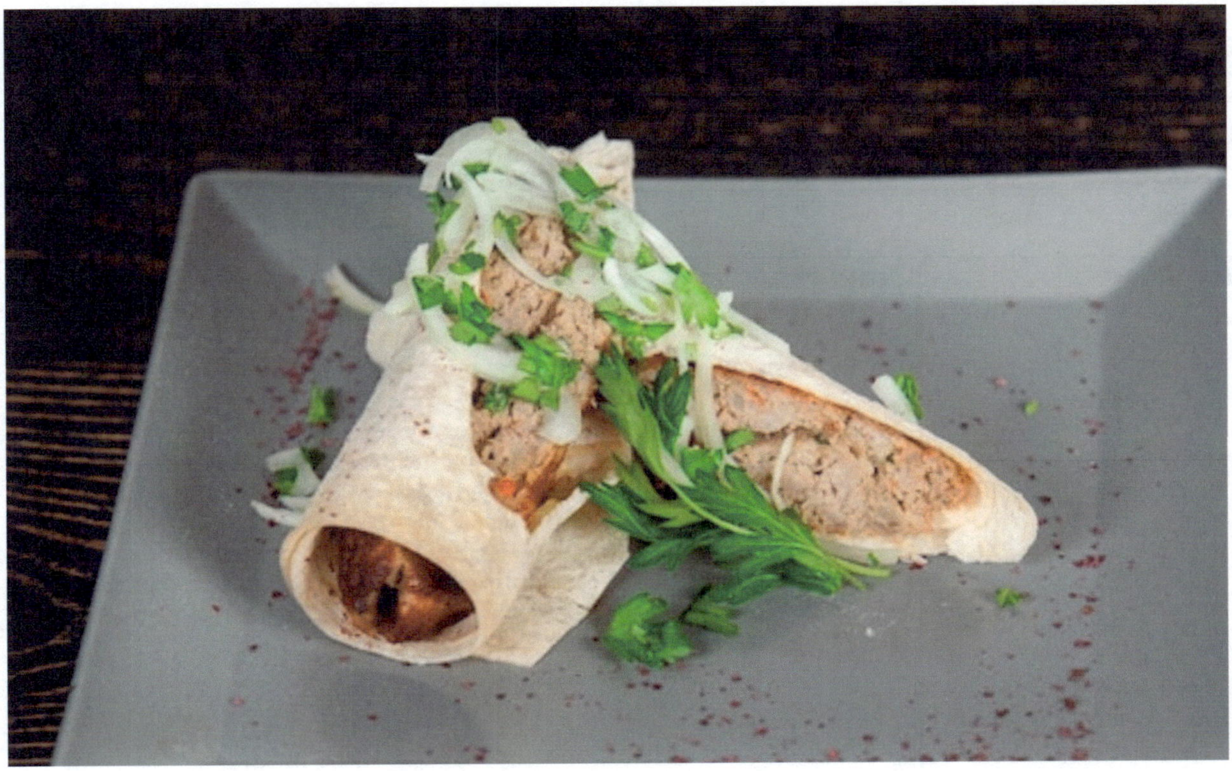

9. Greek Yogurt Chicken Caesar Wrap

Prep.Time: 15 min

Cook Time: 0 min

Serving: 2

Beverage pairing: Iced Tea

Ingredients:

- 2 whole grain wraps
- 1 cup cooked chicken breast, shredded
- 1/4 cup Greek yogurt
- 2 tablespoons grated Parmesan cheese
- 1 tablespoon lemon juice
- 1 teaspoon Dijon mustard
- 1 teaspoon Worcestershire sauce
- 1/2 teaspoon garlic powder
- Salt and pepper to taste
- 2 cups romaine lettuce, chopped

Preparation:

1. In a small bowl, mix together Greek yogurt, Parmesan cheese, lemon juice, Dijon mustard, Worcestershire sauce, garlic powder, salt, and pepper to make the Caesar dressing.
2. Lay out the wraps on a clean surface.
3. Spread Caesar dressing onto each wrap.
4. Top with shredded chicken and chopped romaine lettuce.
5. Roll up the wraps tightly, tucking in the sides as you go.
6. Slice each wrap in half diagonally and serve.

Nutrition Facts (per serving):

- Calories: 320
- Carbohydrates: 25g
- Protein: 30g
- Fat: 12g

10. Shrimp and Broccoli Stir-Fry with Brown Rice

Prep.Time:	Cook Time:	Serving:	Beverage pairing:
20 min	15 min	2	Green Tea

Ingredients:

- 1 cup brown rice, cooked
- 8 oz shrimp, peeled and deveined
- 2 cups broccoli florets
- 1 bell pepper, sliced
- 2 cloves garlic, minced
- 1 tablespoon olive oil
- 2 tablespoons low-sodium soy sauce
- 1 tablespoon honey
- 1 teaspoon grated ginger
- Salt and pepper to taste
- Sesame seeds for garnish (optional)

Preparation:

1. In a small bowl, whisk together soy sauce, honey, grated ginger, salt, and pepper to make the sauce.
2. Heat olive oil in a large skillet over medium-high heat. Add minced garlic and cook for 1 minute.
3. Add shrimp to the skillet and cook for 2-3 minutes per side, until pink and cooked through. Remove shrimp from the skillet and set aside.
4. In the same skillet, add broccoli florets and bell pepper slices. Cook for 4-5 minutes, or until vegetables are tender-crisp.
5. Return cooked shrimp to the skillet, then pour the sauce over the shrimp and vegetables. Stir to coat evenly and cook for an additional 1-2 minutes.
6. Serve shrimp and broccoli stir-fry over cooked brown rice. Garnish with sesame seeds if desired.

Nutritional Information (per serving):

- Calories: 380
- Carbohydrates: 45g
- Protein: 25g
- Fat: 12g

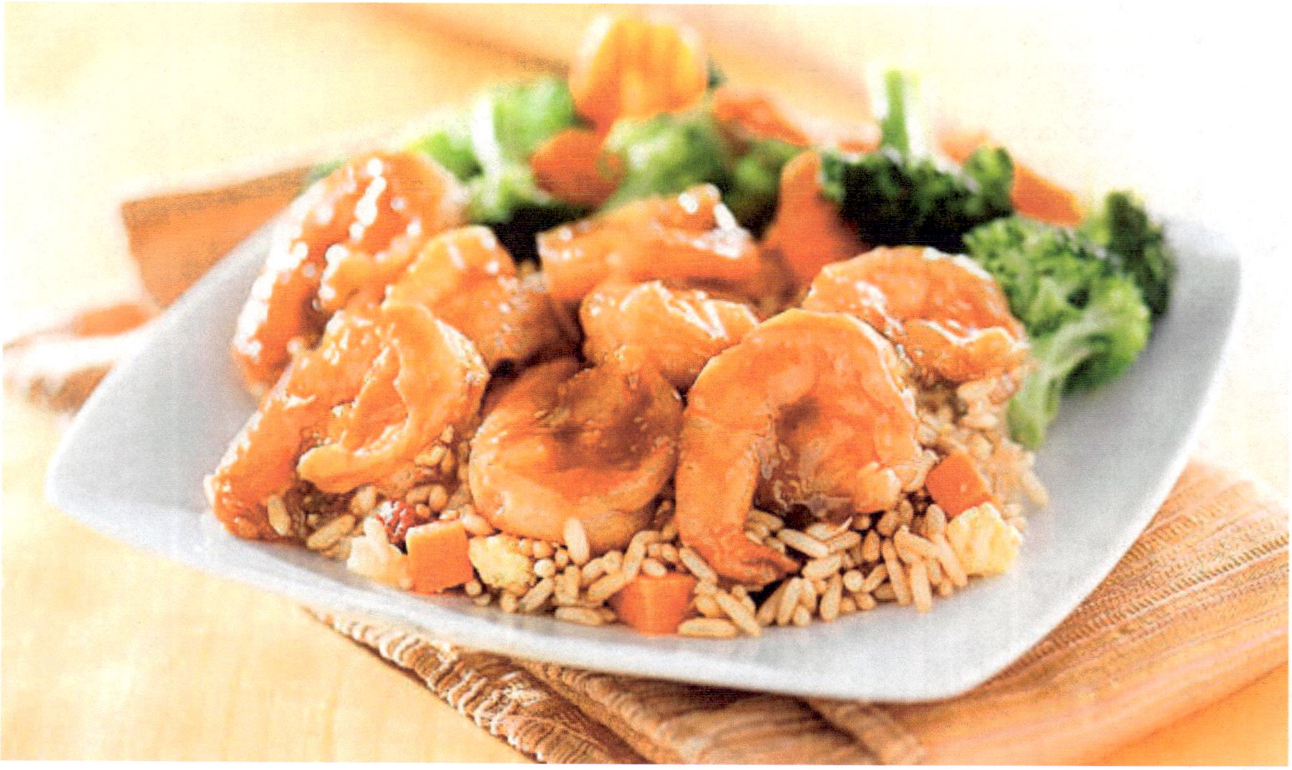

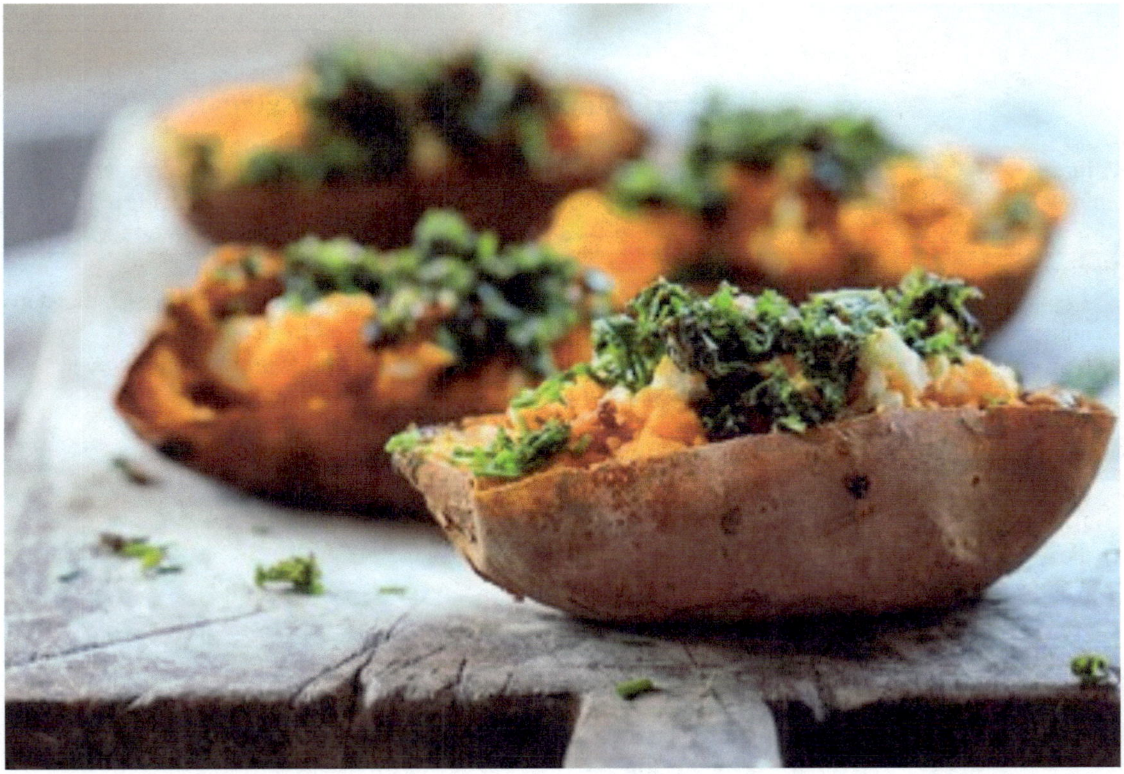

11. Chickpea and Spinach Stuffed Sweet Potatoes

Prep.Time: 10 min

Cook Time: 50 min

Serving: 2

Beverage pairing: Herbal Tea

Ingredients:

- 2 medium sweet potatoes
- 1 can (15 oz) chickpeas, drained and rinsed
- 2 cups fresh spinach leaves
- 1/4 cup diced red onion
- 1 clove garlic, minced
- 1 tablespoon olive oil
- 1 teaspoon ground cumin
- 1/2 teaspoon paprika
- Salt and pepper to taste
- 1/4 cup plain Greek yogurt (optional)

Preparation:

1. Preheat oven to 400°F (200°C).
2. Wash sweet potatoes and pierce them several times with a fork. Place them on a baking sheet and bake for 45-50 minutes, or until tender.
3. Meanwhile, heat olive oil in a skillet over medium heat. Add diced red onion and minced garlic, and cook for 2-3 minutes until softened.
4. Add chickpeas, ground cumin, paprika, salt, and pepper to the skillet. Cook for 5-7 minutes, stirring occasionally, until chickpeas are slightly crispy.
5. Add fresh spinach leaves to the skillet and cook until wilted.
6. Slice open the baked sweet potatoes and fluff the insides with a fork. Divide the chickpea and spinach mixture evenly among the sweet potatoes.
7. Serve stuffed sweet potatoes with a dollop of plain Greek yogurt on top if desired.

Nutrition Facts (per serving):

- Calories: 350
- Carbohydrates: 60g
- Protein: 15g
- Fat: 7g

12. Turkey and Avocado Quinoa Salad

Prep.Time: 15 min

Cook Time: 0 min

Serving: 2

Beverage pairing: Lemonade

Ingredients:

- 1 cup cooked quinoa
- 6 oz cooked turkey breast, diced
- 1 avocado, diced
- 1/4 cup cherry tomatoes, halved
- 1/4 cup cucumber, diced
- 2 tablespoons chopped fresh cilantro
- Juice of 1 lime
- Salt and pepper to taste

Preparation:

1. In a large bowl, combine cooked quinoa, diced turkey breast, diced avocado, cherry tomatoes, cucumber, and chopped fresh cilantro.
2. Squeeze lime juice over the salad and toss gently to combine.
3. Season with salt and pepper to taste before serving.

Nutritional Information (per serving):

- Calories: 380
- Carbohydrates: 25g
- Protein: 30g
- Fat: 18g

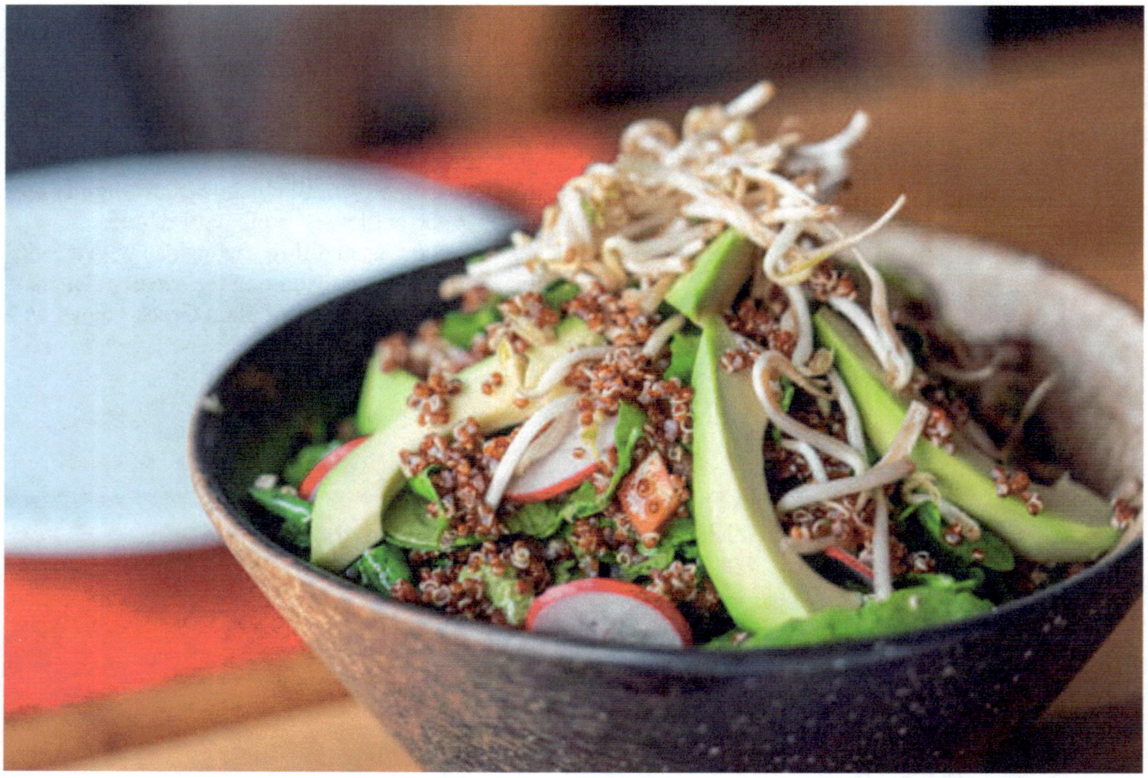

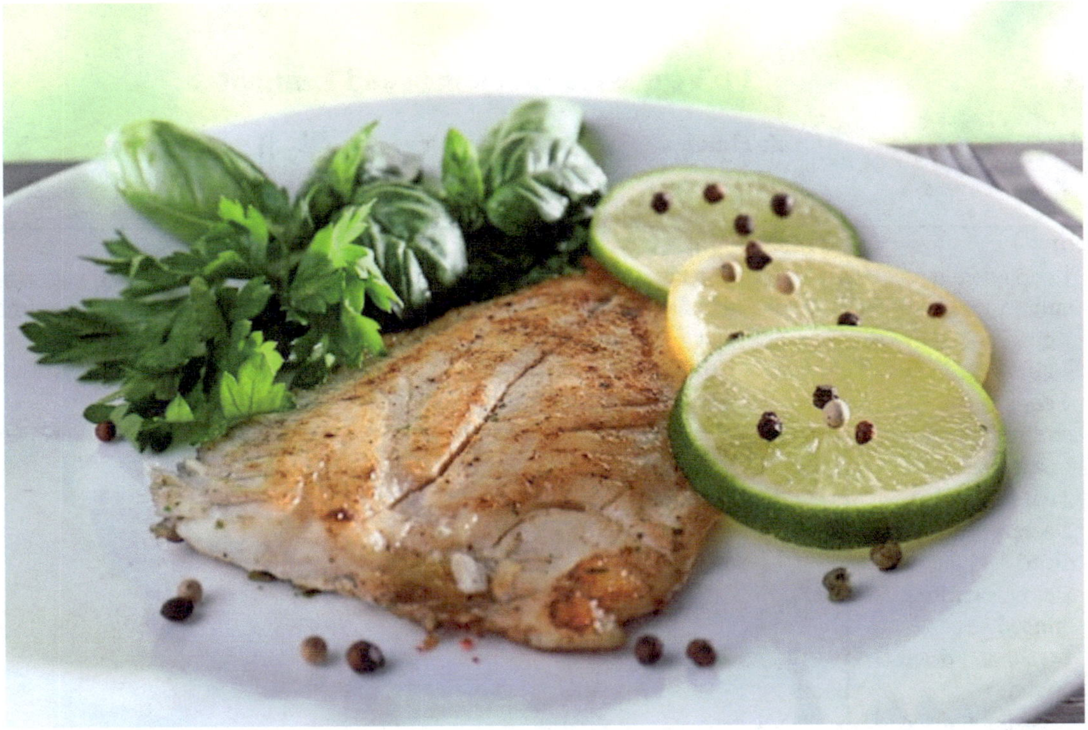

13. Baked Cod with Lemon and Herbs

Prep.Time:	**Cook Time:**	**Serving:**	**Beverage pairing:**
10 min	15 min	2	Herbal Tea

Ingredients:

- 2 cod fillets (about 6 oz each)
- 1 tablespoon olive oil
- 1 tablespoon fresh lemon juice
- 1 teaspoon chopped fresh dill
- 1 teaspoon chopped fresh parsley
- Salt and pepper to taste
- Lemon wedges for serving

Preparation:

1. Preheat oven to 400°F (200°C).
2. Place cod fillets on a baking sheet lined with parchment paper.
3. In a small bowl, mix together olive oil, lemon juice, chopped dill, chopped parsley, salt, and pepper.
4. Brush the mixture over the cod fillets, coating them evenly.
5. Bake for 12-15 minutes, or until fish is cooked through and flakes easily with a fork.
6. Serve baked cod with lemon wedges on the side.

Nutrition Facts (per serving):

- Calories: 250
- Carbohydrates: 1g
- Protein: 30g
- Fat: 13g

14. Veggie-loaded Quinoa and Lentil Stew

Prep.Time: 15 min

Cook Time: 30 min

Serving: 4

Beverage pairing: Herbal Tea

Ingredients:

- 1 cup cooked quinoa
- 1 cup cooked green lentils
- 4 cups vegetable broth
- 1 onion, diced
- 2 carrots, diced
- 2 celery stalks, diced
- 2 cloves garlic, minced
- 1 teaspoon dried thyme
- 1 teaspoon dried rosemary
- 1 can (15 oz) diced tomatoes
- 2 cups chopped kale leaves
- Salt and pepper to taste

Preparation:

1. In a large pot, combine cooked quinoa, cooked green lentils, vegetable broth, diced onion, carrots, celery, minced garlic, dried thyme, dried rosemary, and diced tomatoes.
2. Bring to a boil, then reduce heat and simmer for 20-25 minutes, or until vegetables are tender.
3. Stir in chopped kale leaves and cook for an additional 2-3 minutes until wilted.
4. Season with salt and pepper to taste before serving.

Nutritional Information (per serving):

- Calories: 280
- Carbohydrates: 45g
- Protein: 15g
- Fat: 3g

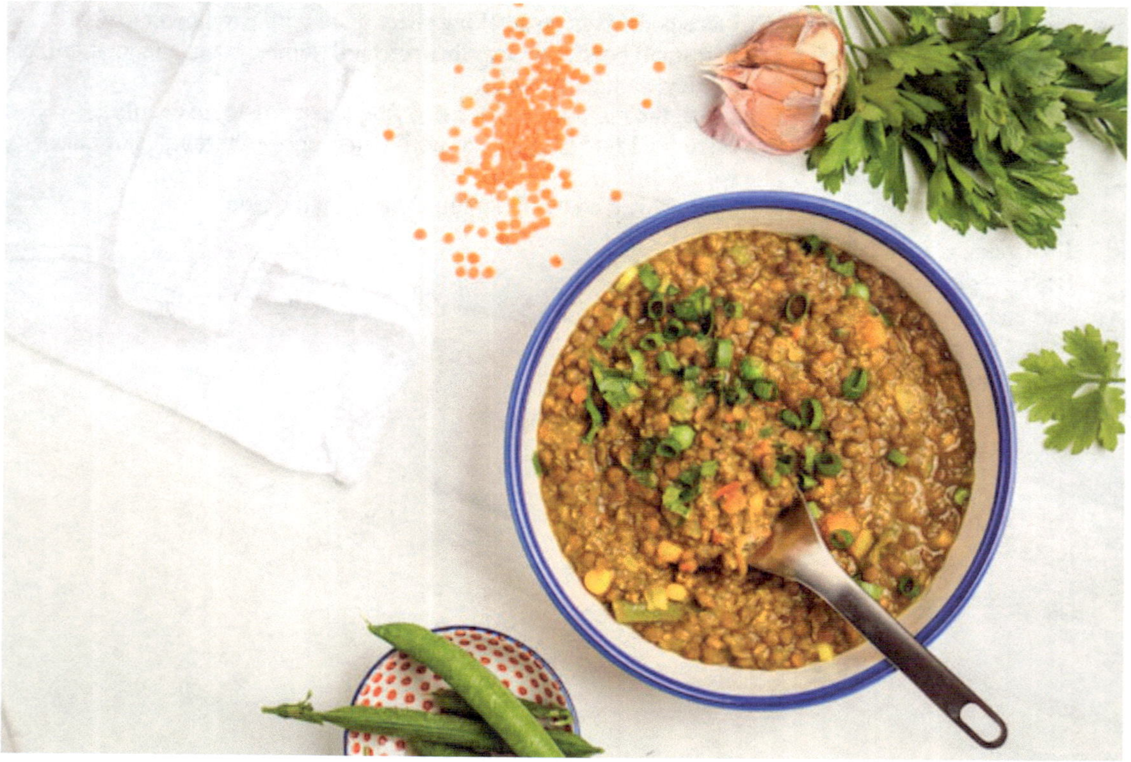

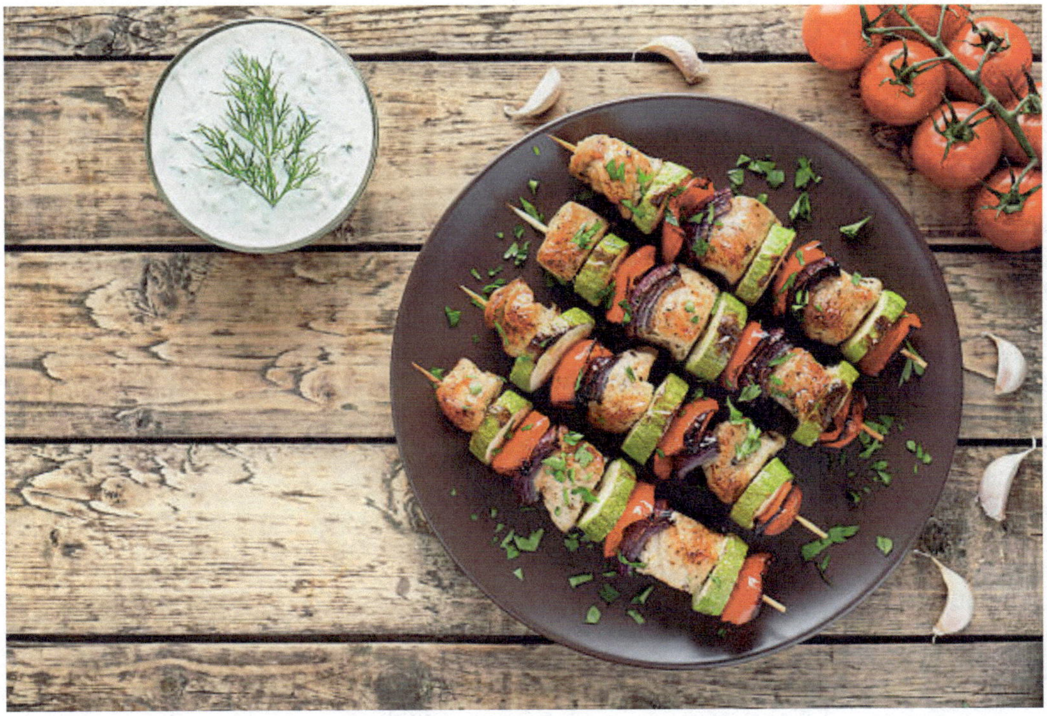

15. Chicken and Vegetable Skewers with Tzatziki Sauce

Prep.Time: 20 min | **Cook Time:** 12 min | **Serving:** 2 | **Beverage pairing:** Iced Tea

Ingredients:

- 2 boneless, skinless chicken breasts, cut into chunks
- 1 bell pepper, cut into chunks
- 1 zucchini, sliced
- 1 onion, cut into chunks
- 8 cherry tomatoes
- 1 teaspoon oregano
- Salt and pepper to taste
- Wooden skewers, soaked in water for 30 minutes
- 1/2 cup plain Greek yogurt
- 1/2 cucumber, grated and squeezed to remove excess moisture
- 1 tablespoon chopped fresh dill

Preparation:

1. Preheat grill to medium-high heat.
2. Thread chicken chunks, bell pepper chunks, zucchini slices, onion chunks, and cherry tomatoes onto soaked wooden skewers, alternating ingredients.
3. In a small bowl, whisk together olive oil, dried oregano, salt, and pepper. Brush the mixture over the skewers.
4. Grill skewers for 10-12 minutes, turning occasionally, until chicken is cooked through and vegetables are tender.
5. Meanwhile, prepare the Tzatziki sauce by combining Greek yogurt, grated cucumber, minced garlic, chopped dill, lemon juice, salt, and pepper in a bowl. Stir well to combine.
6. Serve grilled chicken and vegetable skewers with Tzatziki sauce on the side.

Nutrition Facts (per serving):

- Calories: 320
- Carbohydrates: 15g
- Protein: 30g
- Fat: 15g

16. Zucchini Noodles with Pesto and Cherry Tomatoes

Prep.Time: 10 min

Cook Time: 5 min

Serving: 2

Beverage pairing: Lemonade

Ingredients:

- 2 medium zucchinis, spiralized into noodles
- 1/2 cup cherry tomatoes, halved
- 1/4 cup pesto sauce (homemade or store-bought)
- Salt and pepper to taste
- Grated Parmesan cheese for garnish (optional)

Preparation:

1. Heat a large skillet over medium heat.
2. Add zucchini noodles to the skillet and cook for 2-3 minutes, stirring occasionally, until slightly softened.
3. Stir in cherry tomatoes and pesto sauce. Cook for an additional 1-2 minutes, until heated through.
4. Season with salt and pepper to taste.
5. Serve zucchini noodles with pesto and cherry tomatoes, garnished with grated Parmesan cheese if desired.

Nutritional Information (per serving):

- Calories: 180
- Carbohydrates: 10g
- Protein: 5g
- Fat: 15g

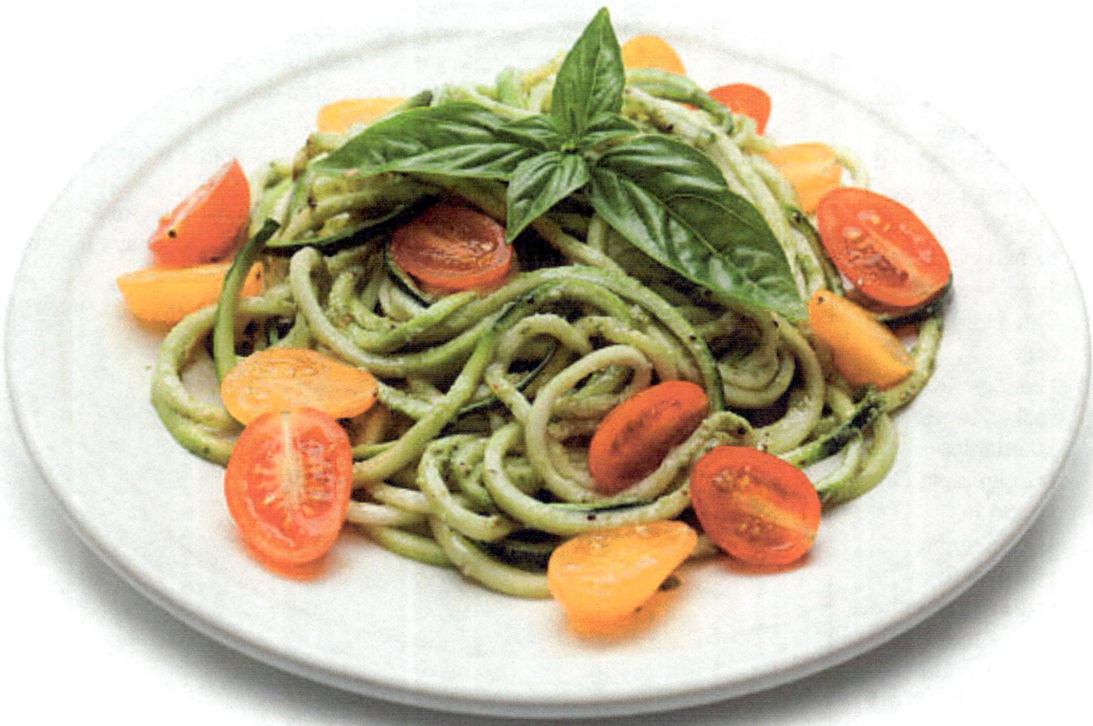

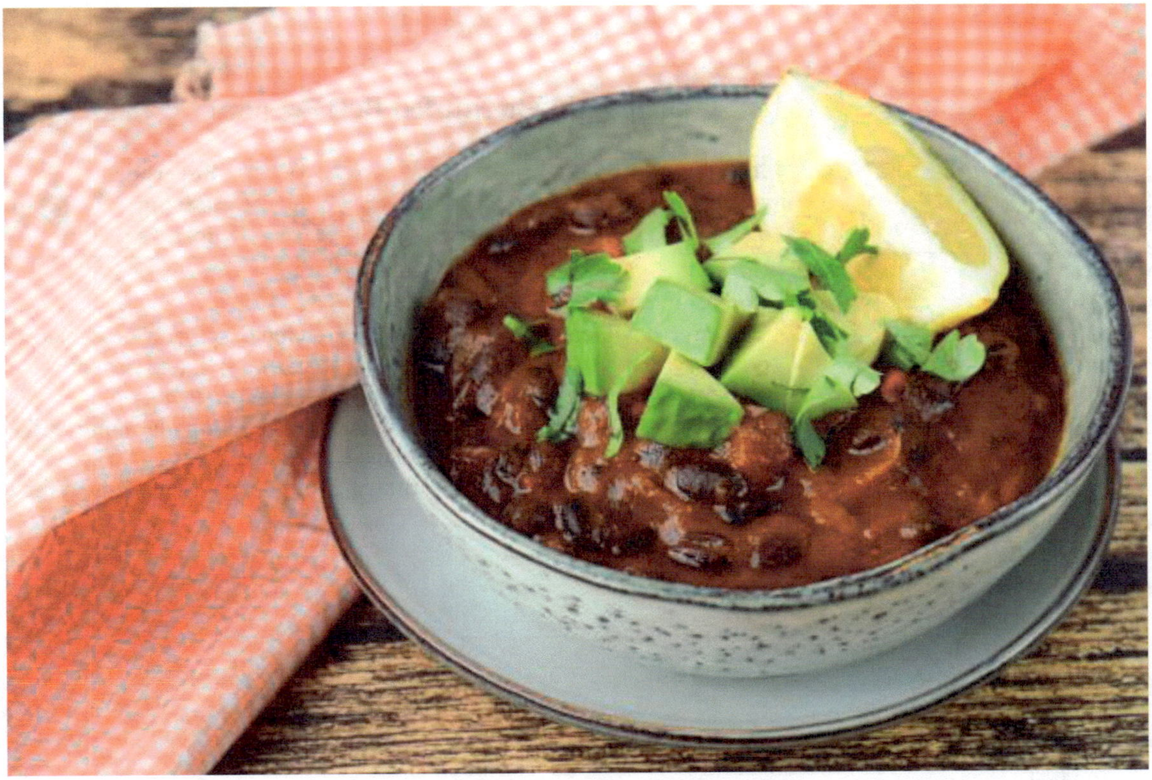

17. Turkey Chili with Black Beans and Tomatoes

Prep.Time: 10 min

Cook Time: 30 min

Serving: 3

Beverage pairing: Iced Tea

Ingredients:

- 2 boneless, skinless chicken breasts, cut into chunks
- 1 bell pepper, cut into chunks
- 1 zucchini, sliced
- 1 onion, cut into chunks
- 8 cherry tomatoes
- 1 teaspoon oregano
- Salt and pepper to taste
- Wooden skewers, soaked in water for 30 minutes
- 1/2 cup plain Greek yogurt
- 1/2 cucumber, grated and squeezed to remove excess moisture
- 1 tablespoon chopped fresh dill

Preparation:

1. In a large pot, cook ground turkey over medium heat until browned.
2. Add diced onion and minced garlic to the pot. Cook for 2-3 minutes until onion is translucent.
3. Stir in black beans, diced tomatoes, chicken broth, chili powder, ground cumin, paprika, salt, and pepper.
4. Bring chili to a boil, then reduce heat and simmer for 20-25 minutes, stirring occasionally.
5. Serve turkey chili hot, garnished with chopped fresh cilantro if desired.

Nutrition Facts (per serving):

- Calories: 320
- Carbohydrates: 25g
- Protein: 30g
- Fat: 10g

18. Spinach and Feta Stuffed Bell Peppers

Prep.Time: 15 min

Cook Time: 35 min

Serving: 2

Beverage pairing: Iced Tea

Ingredients:

- 2 bell peppers, halved and seeds removed
- 1 cup cooked quinoa
- 1 cup chopped fresh spinach
- 1/2 cup crumbled feta cheese
- 2 tablespoons chopped fresh parsley
- 1 tablespoon olive oil
- 1 clove garlic, minced
- Salt and pepper to taste

Preparation:

1. Preheat oven to 375°F (190°C).
2. In a large bowl, combine cooked quinoa, chopped spinach, crumbled feta cheese, chopped parsley, olive oil, minced garlic, salt, and pepper.
3. Stuff each bell pepper half with the quinoa mixture.
4. Place stuffed bell peppers in a baking dish. Cover with aluminum foil and bake for 25-30 minutes, or until peppers are tender.
5. Remove foil and bake for an additional 5 minutes to lightly brown the tops.
6. Serve spinach and feta stuffed bell peppers hot.

Nutritional Information (per serving):

- Calories: 220
- Carbohydrates: 20g
- Protein: 8g
- Fat: 12g

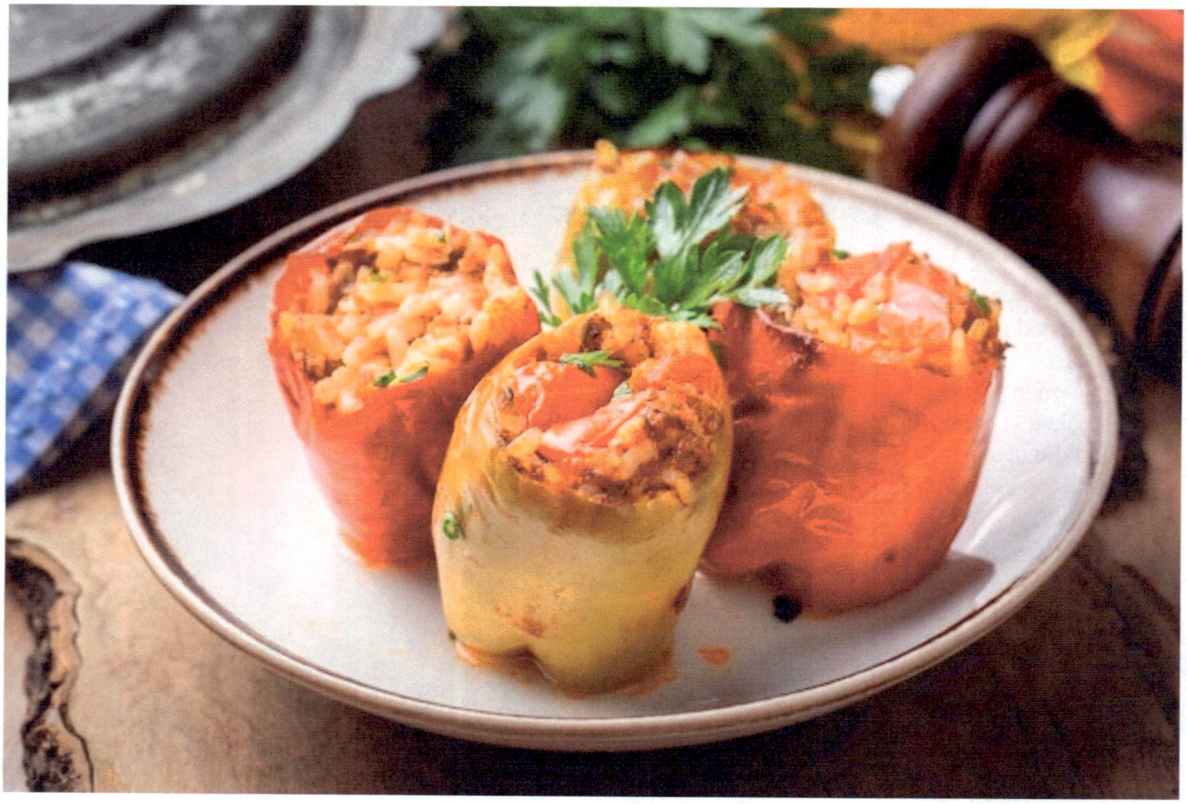

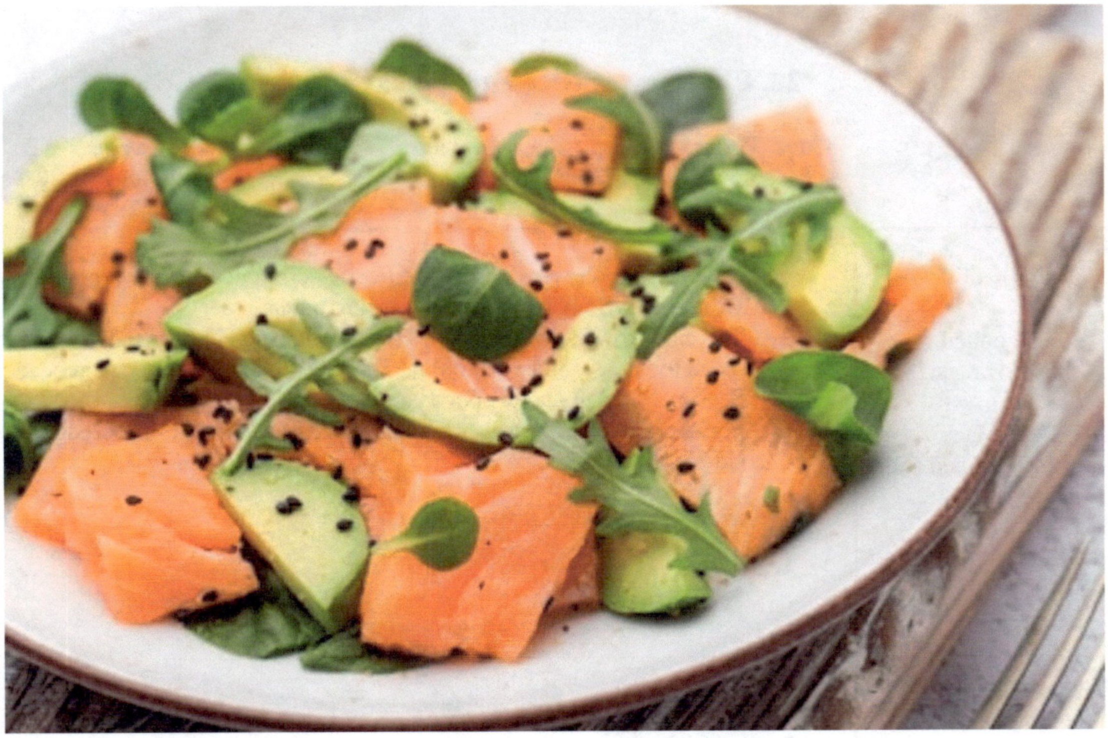

19. Asian-style Salmon Salad with Sesame Ginger Dressing

Prep.Time: 10 min

Cook Time: 15 min

Serving: 2

Beverage pairing: Green Tea

Ingredients:

- 2 salmon fillets (about 6 oz each)
- 4 cups mixed salad greens
- 1/2 cucumber, sliced
- 1/4 cup shredded carrots
- 1/4 cup sliced radishes
- 2 tablespoons chopped fresh cilantro
- 1 tablespoon sesame seeds
- 2 tablespoons rice vinegar
- 1 tablespoon soy sauce
- 1 tablespoon sesame oil
- 1 teaspoon grated ginger
- 1 teaspoon honey

Preparation:

1. Preheat oven to 400°F (200°C).
2. Place salmon fillets on a baking sheet lined with parchment paper. Season with salt and pepper.
3. Bake salmon for 12-15 minutes, or until cooked through and flakes easily with a fork.
4. In a small bowl, whisk together rice vinegar, soy sauce, sesame oil, grated ginger, honey, salt, and pepper to make the dressing.
5. In a large salad bowl, combine mixed salad greens, sliced cucumber, shredded carrots, sliced radishes, chopped cilantro, and sesame seeds.
6. Divide salad among plates, top with baked salmon fillets, and drizzle with sesame ginger dressing.

Nutrition Facts (per serving):

- Calories: 350
- Carbohydrates: 15g
- Protein: 30g
- Fat: 20g

20. Cauliflower Rice and Chicken Burrito Bowl

Prep.Time: 10 min | **Cook Time:** 0 min | **Serving:** 2 | **Beverage pairing:** Iced Tea

Ingredients:

- 2 cups cauliflower rice
- 1 cup cooked chicken breast, diced
- 1/2 cup black beans, drained and rinsed
- 1/2 cup corn kernels
- 1/4 cup diced tomatoes
- 1/4 cup diced red onion
- 1/4 cup chopped fresh cilantro
- 1/2 avocado, diced
- 1 lime, cut into wedges
- Salt and pepper to taste

Preparation:

1. Heat cauliflower rice in a skillet over medium heat until warmed through.
2. Divide cauliflower rice among serving bowls.
3. Top cauliflower rice with diced chicken breast, black beans, corn kernels, diced tomatoes, diced red onion, chopped cilantro, and diced avocado.
4. Season with salt and pepper to taste.
5. Serve cauliflower rice and chicken burrito bowls with lime wedges on the side.

Nutritional Information (per serving):

- Calories: 320
- Carbohydrates: 25g
- Protein: 25g
- Fat: 15g

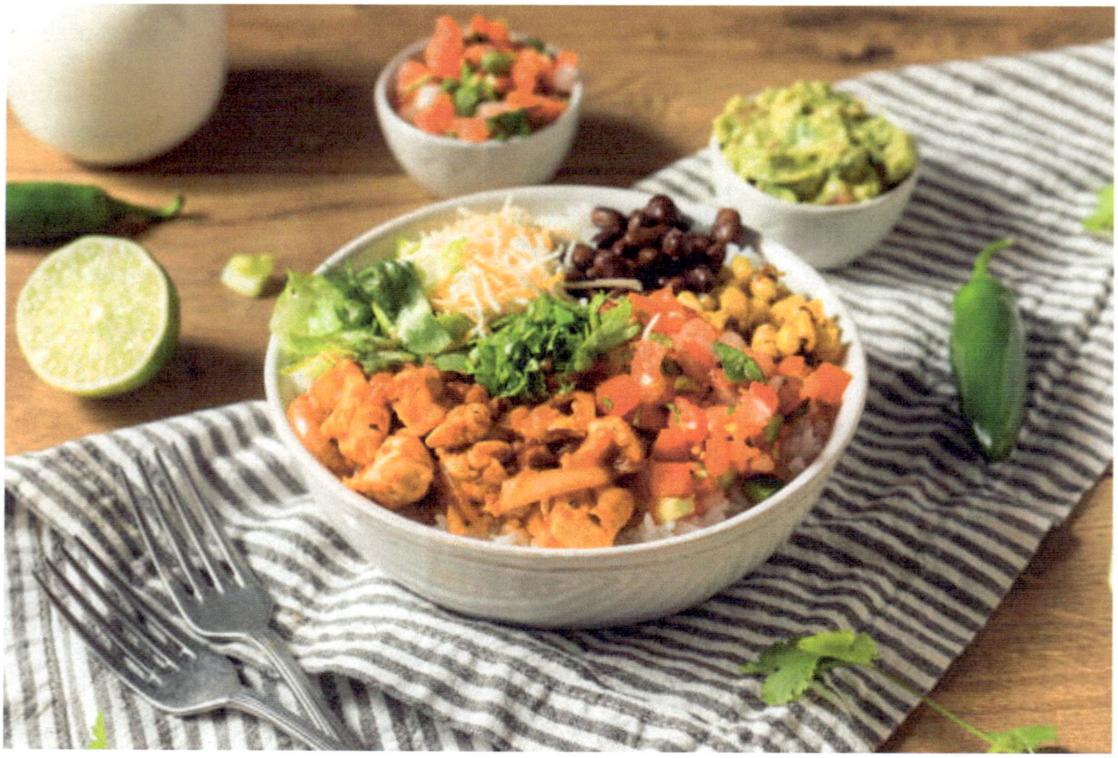

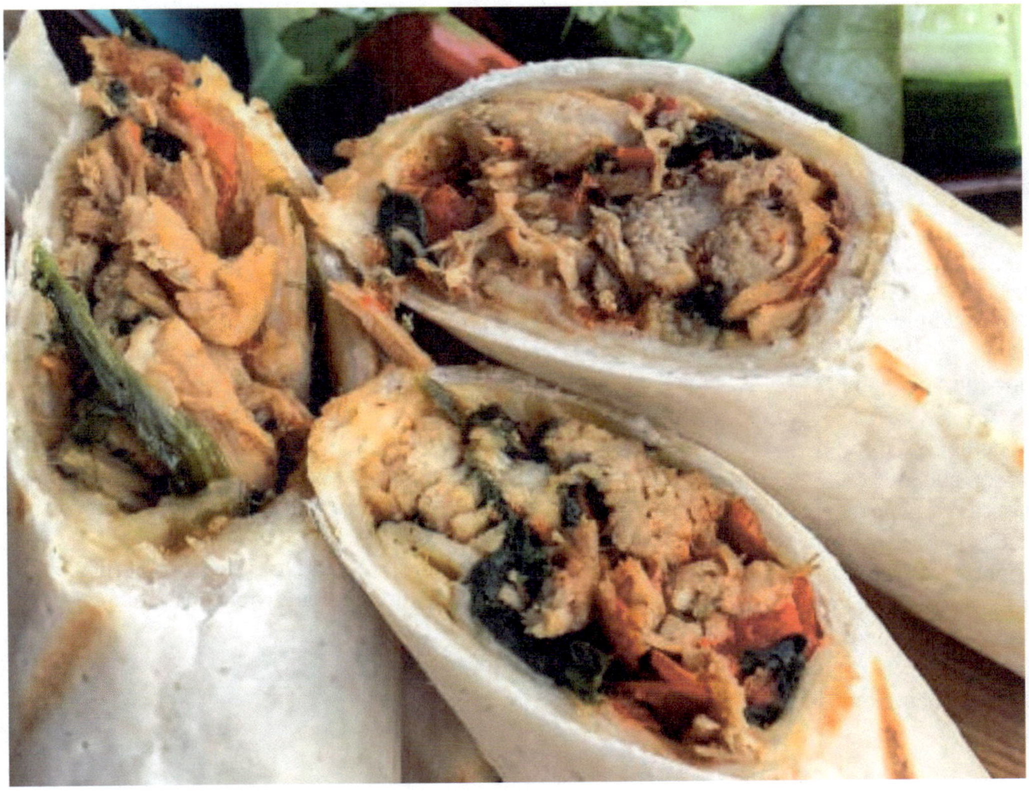

21. Beef and Vegetable Lettuce Wraps

Prep.Time: 15 min

Cook Time: 15 min

Serving: 4

Beverage pairing: Iced Tea

Ingredients:

- 8 large lettuce leaves (such as butter or iceberg lettuce)
- 1/2 lb lean ground beef
- 1/2 cup diced bell peppers
- 1/4 cup diced onion
- 2 cloves garlic, minced
- 2 tablespoons low-sodium soy sauce
- 1 tablespoon hoisin sauce
- 1 teaspoon sesame oil
- 1 teaspoon grated ginger
- 1/4 cup chopped green onions
- 1/4 cup chopped fresh cilantro

Preparation:

1. Heat a large skillet over medium-high heat.
2. Add ground beef to the skillet and cook until browned, breaking it apart with a spoon.
3. Add diced bell peppers, diced onion, and minced garlic to the skillet. Cook for 3-4 minutes until vegetables are tender.
4. In a small bowl, whisk together soy sauce, hoisin sauce, sesame oil, and grated ginger. Pour the sauce over the beef and vegetable mixture in the skillet.
5. Stir in chopped green onions and chopped cilantro. Cook for an additional 1-2 minutes.
6. Spoon the beef and vegetable mixture onto lettuce leaves.
7. Serve beef and vegetable lettuce wraps immediately.

Nutrition Facts (per serving):

- Calories: 250
- Carbohydrates: 10g
- Protein: 20g
- Fat: 15g

22. Grilled Eggplant and Hummus Sandwich

Prep.Time: 10 min | **Cook Time:** 8 min | **Serving:** 2 | **Beverage pairing:** Iced Tea

Ingredients:

- 4 slices whole grain bread
- 1 medium eggplant, sliced
- 1/4 cup hummus
- 1/4 cup sliced roasted red peppers
- 2 tablespoons chopped fresh parsley
- 1 tablespoon olive oil
- Salt and pepper to taste

Preparation:

1. Preheat grill or grill pan over medium-high heat.
2. Brush eggplant slices with olive oil and season with salt and pepper.
3. Grill eggplant slices for 3-4 minutes per side, or until tender and grill marks appear.
4. Toast slices of whole grain bread.
5. Spread hummus evenly onto each slice of bread.
6. Layer grilled eggplant slices, sliced roasted red peppers, and chopped fresh parsley onto two slices of bread.
7. Top with the remaining slices of bread to make sandwiches.
8. Serve grilled eggplant and hummus sandwiches immediately.

Nutritional Information (per serving):

- Calories: 280
- Carbohydrates: 35g
- Protein: 8g
- Fat: 12g

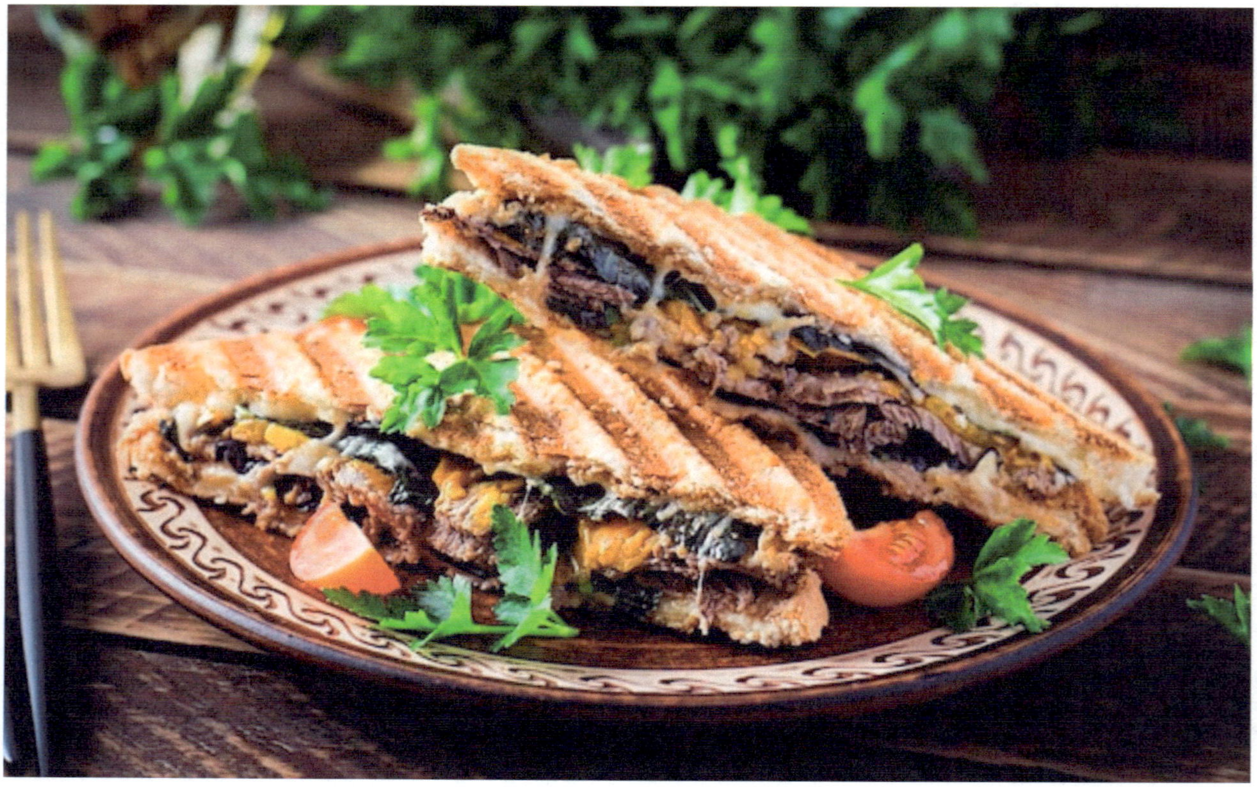

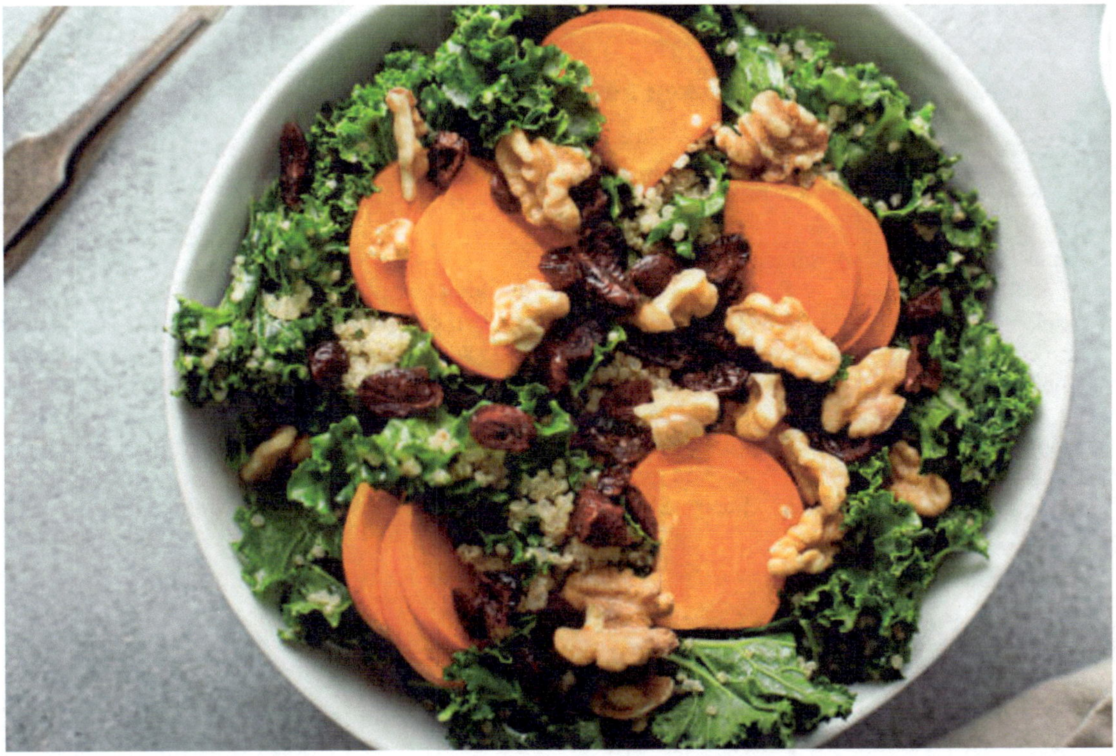

23. Quinoa and Kale Salad with Cranberries and Walnuts

Prep.Time: 10 min

Cook Time: 0 min

Serving: 2

Beverage pairing: Iced Tea

Ingredients:

- 1 cup cooked quinoa
- 2 cups chopped kale leaves
- 1/4 cup dried cranberries
- 1/4 cup chopped walnuts
- 2 tablespoons olive oil
- 1 tablespoon balsamic vinegar
- 1 teaspoon honey
- Salt and pepper to taste

Preparation:

1. In a large bowl, combine cooked quinoa, chopped kale leaves, dried cranberries, and chopped walnuts.
2. In a small bowl, whisk together olive oil, balsamic vinegar, honey, salt, and pepper to make the dressing.
3. Pour the dressing over the salad and toss until evenly coated.
4. Serve quinoa and kale salad immediately.

Nutrition Facts (per serving):

- Calories: 300
- Carbohydrates: 30g
- Protein: 8g
- Fat: 18g

24. Chicken and Vegetable Kebabs with Quinoa

Prep.Time: 20 min

Cook Time: 12 min

Serving: 2

Beverage pairing: Iced Tea

Ingredients:

- 2 boneless, skinless chicken breasts, cut into chunks
- 1 bell pepper, cut into chunks
- 1 zucchini, sliced
- 1 onion, cut into chunks
- 8 cherry tomatoes
- 2 tablespoons olive oil
- 1 teaspoon dried oregano
- Salt and pepper to taste
- Wooden skewers, soaked in water for 30 minutes
- 1 cup cooked quinoa

Preparation:

1. Preheat grill to medium-high heat.
2. Thread chicken chunks, bell pepper chunks, zucchini slices, onion chunks, and cherry tomatoes onto soaked wooden skewers, alternating ingredients.
3. In a small bowl, whisk together olive oil, dried oregano, salt, and pepper. Brush the mixture over the skewers.
4. Grill skewers for 10-12 minutes, turning occasionally, until chicken is cooked through and vegetables are tender.
5. Serve chicken and vegetable kebabs with cooked quinoa.

Nutritional Information (per serving):

- Calories: 350
- Carbohydrates: 30g
- Protein: 30g
- Fat: 15g

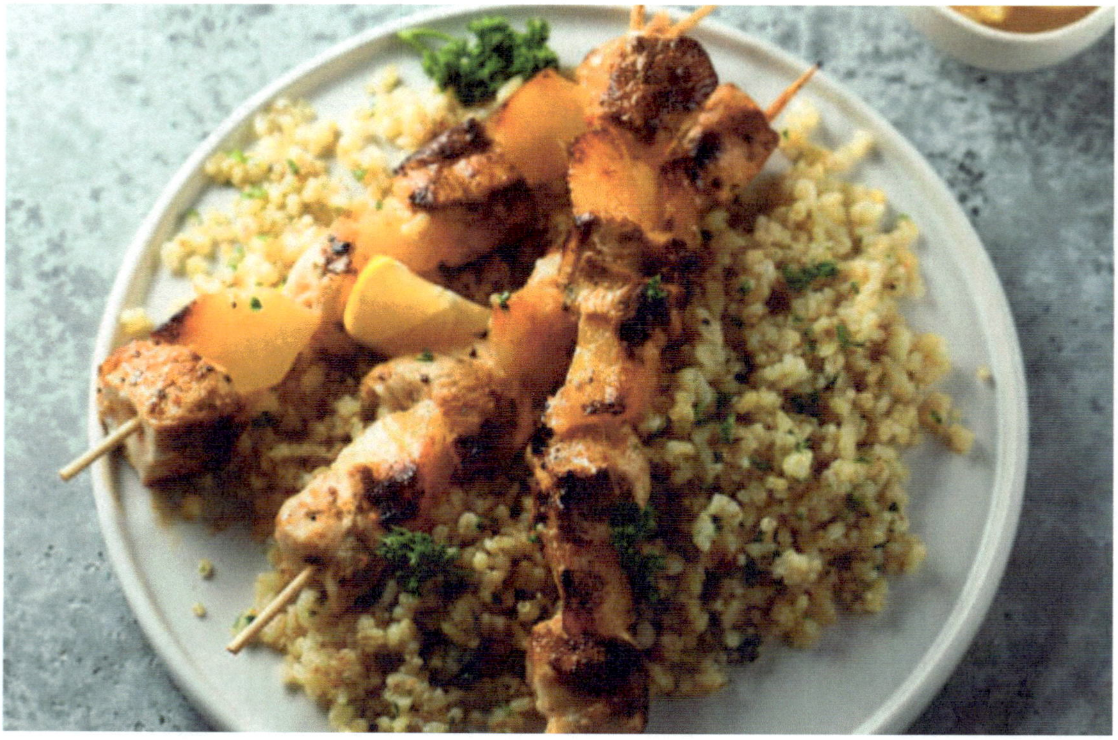

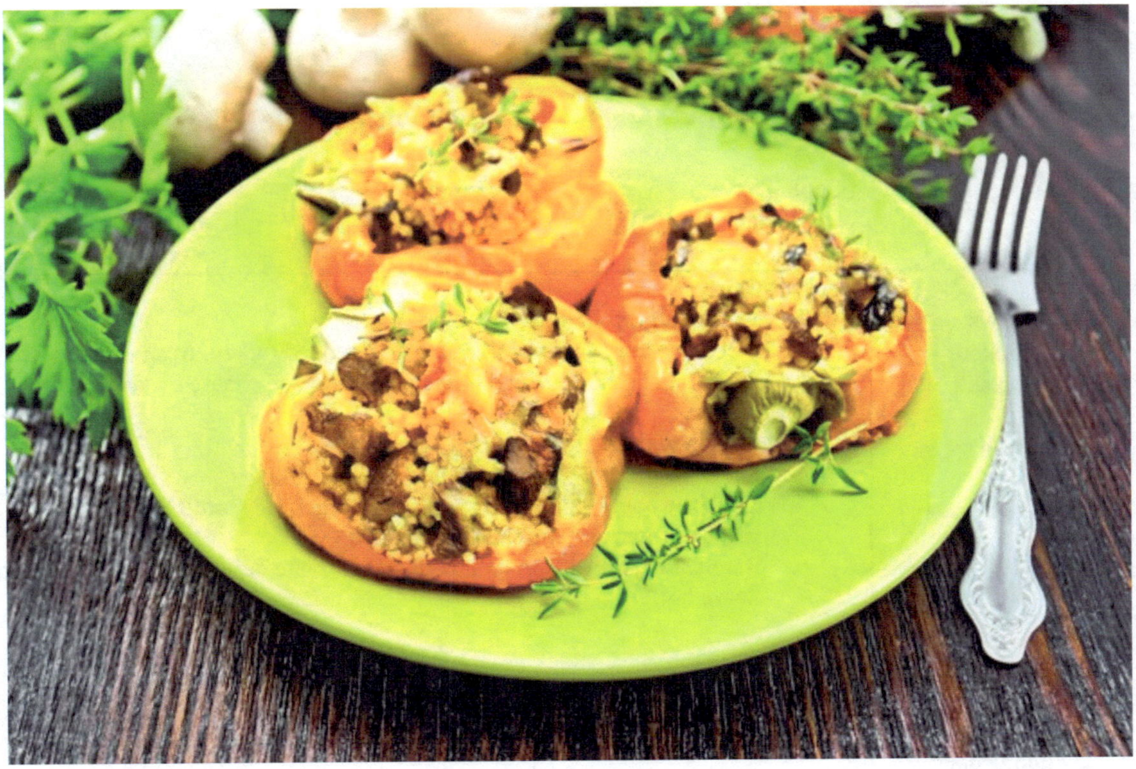

25. Lentil and Mushroom Stuffed Bell Peppers

Prep.Time: 15 min

Cook Time: 30 min

Serving: 2

Beverage pairing: lemonade

Ingredients:

- 2 large bell peppers, halved and seeds removed
- 1 cup cooked lentils
- 1 cup diced mushrooms
- 1/2 cup diced onion
- 2 cloves garlic, minced
- 1/2 cup diced tomatoes
- 1/4 cup chopped fresh parsley
- 1 teaspoon dried oregano
- Salt and pepper to taste
- Grated Parmesan cheese for topping (optional)

Preparation:

1. Preheat oven to 375°F (190°C).
2. In a skillet, heat a tablespoon of olive oil over medium heat. Add diced onion and minced garlic, cook until softened.
3. Add diced mushrooms and cook until they release their moisture and start to brown.
4. Stir in cooked lentils, diced tomatoes, chopped parsley, dried oregano, salt, and pepper. Cook for another 2-3 minutes.
5. Place bell pepper halves in a baking dish. Spoon the lentil and mushroom mixture evenly into each pepper half.
6. Cover the dish with aluminum foil and bake for 25-30 minutes, until peppers are tender.
7. Optionally, sprinkle grated Parmesan cheese over the stuffed peppers before serving.

Nutrition Facts (per serving):

- Calories: 180
- Carbohydrates: 30g
- Protein: 10g
- Fat: 2g

26. Turkey and Spinach Quesadilla with Whole Wheat Toast

Prep.Time: 10 min

Cook Time: 10 min

Serving: 2

Beverage pairing: Iced Tea

Ingredients:

- 2 whole wheat toast
- 1 cup cooked turkey breast, shredded
- 1 cup fresh spinach leaves
- 1/2 cup shredded cheese (such as cheddar or mozzarella)
- 1/4 cup diced tomatoes
- 1/4 cup diced red onion
- Salt and pepper to taste
- Cooking spray or olive oil for cooking

Preparation:

1. Heat a large skillet over medium heat.
2. Place one toast in the skillet. Layer shredded turkey, fresh spinach leaves, diced tomatoes, diced red onion, and shredded cheese evenly over the tortilla.
3. Season with salt and pepper to taste.
4. Place the second toast on top to cover the filling.
5. Cook the quesadilla for 2-3 minutes on each side, until the tortillas are golden brown and the cheese is melted.
6. Remove from heat and let it cool for a minute before slicing into wedges.
7. Serve hot.

Nutritional Information (per serving):

- Calories: 350
- Carbohydrates: 25g
- Protein: 30g
- Fat: 15g

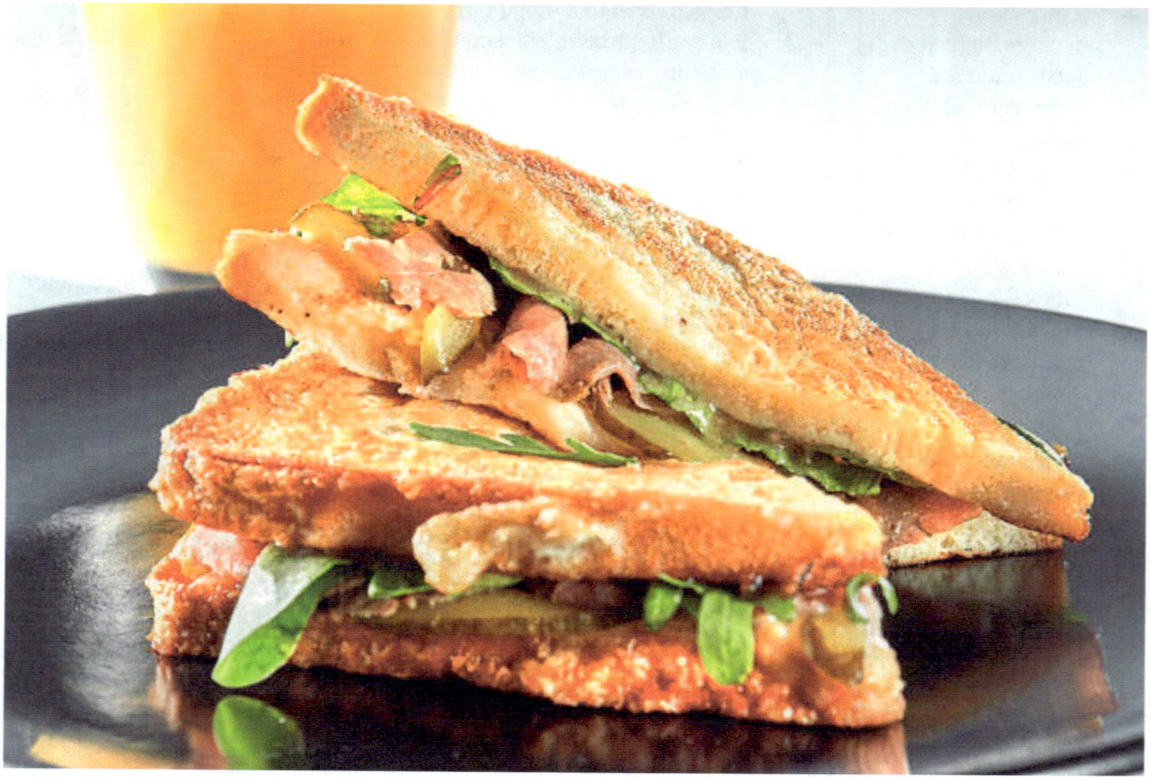

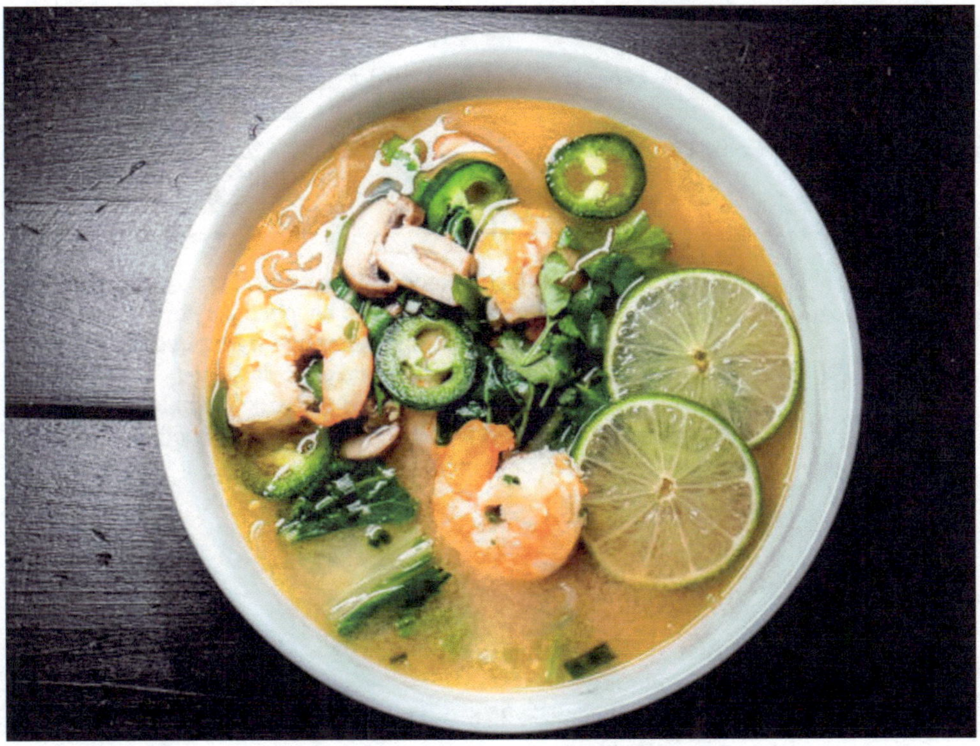

27. Lemon Garlic Shrimp and Broccoli Bowl

Prep.Time: 10 min

Cook Time: 15 min

Serving: 2

Beverage pairing: Herbal Tea

Ingredients:

- 8 oz shrimp, peeled and deveined
- 2 cups broccoli florets
- 2 cloves garlic, minced
- 1 tablespoon olive oil
- 1 tablespoon lemon juice
- Zest of 1 lemon
- Salt and pepper to taste
- Cooked brown rice or quinoa for serving

Preparation:

1. Heat olive oil in a large skillet over medium heat.
2. Add minced garlic and cook for 1 minute until fragrant.
3. Add shrimp to the skillet and cook for 2-3 minutes per side until pink and cooked through.
4. Remove shrimp from the skillet and set aside.
5. In the same skillet, add broccoli florets. Cook for 4-5 minutes, stirring occasionally, until tender-crisp.
6. Return cooked shrimp to the skillet. Add lemon juice and lemon zest. Stir to combine and heat through.
7. Season with salt and pepper to taste.
8. Serve lemon garlic shrimp and broccoli over cooked brown rice or quinoa.

Nutrition Facts (per serving without rice/quinoa):

- Calories: 180
- Carbohydrates: 8g
- Protein: 25g
- Fat: 6g

28. Greek Chickpea and Cucumber Salad

Prep.Time: 10 min

Cook Time: 0 min

Serving: 2

Beverage pairing: Iced Tea

Ingredients:

- 1 can (15 oz) chickpeas, drained and rinsed
- 1 cucumber, diced
- 1/2 cup cherry tomatoes, halved
- 1/4 cup diced red onion
- 1/4 cup Kalamata olives, pitted and halved
- 2 tablespoons chopped fresh parsley
- 2 tablespoons crumbled feta cheese
- 2 tablespoons extra virgin olive oil
- 1 tablespoon red wine vinegar
- 1 teaspoon dried oregano
- Salt and pepper to taste

Preparation:

1. In a large bowl, combine chickpeas, diced cucumber, cherry tomatoes, diced red onion, Kalamata olives, and chopped parsley.
2. In a small bowl, whisk together extra virgin olive oil, red wine vinegar, dried oregano, salt, and pepper to make the dressing.
3. Pour the dressing over the salad and toss to combine.
4. Sprinkle crumbled feta cheese over the salad before serving.
5. Serve chilled or at room temperature.

Nutritional Information (per serving):

- Calories: 280
- Carbohydrates: 25g
- Protein: 9g
- Fat: 16g

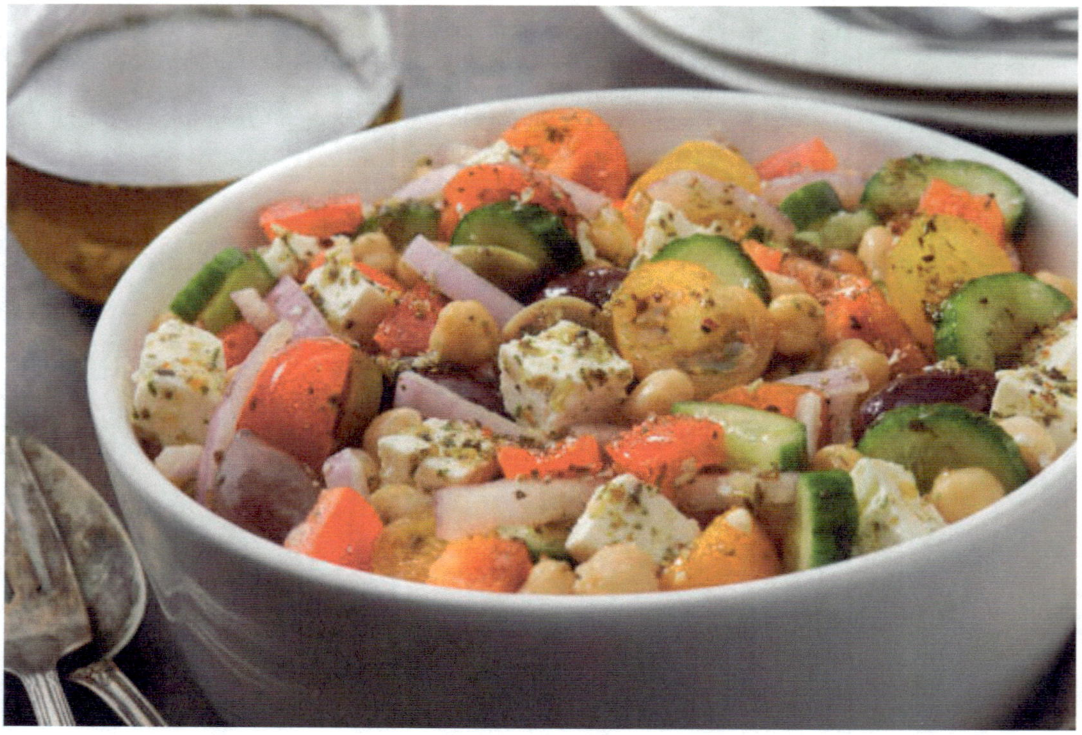

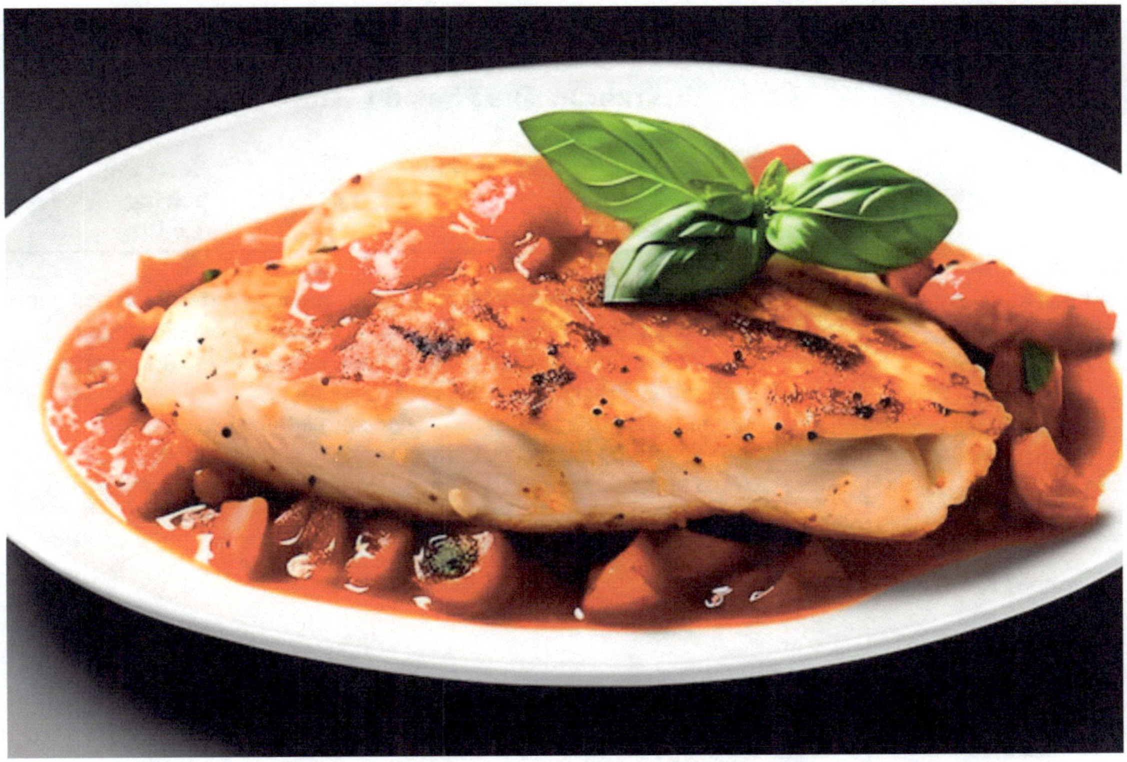

29. Baked Chicken Breast with Tomato Basil Relish

Prep.Time: 10 min

Cook Time: 25 min

Serving: 2

Beverage pairing: Lemonade

Ingredients:

- 2 boneless, skinless chicken breasts
- 1 cup cherry tomatoes, halved
- 2 tablespoons chopped fresh basil
- 1 tablespoon balsamic vinegar
- 1 tablespoon extra virgin olive oil
- 1 clove garlic, minced
- Salt and pepper to taste

Preparation:

1. Preheat oven to 400°F (200°C).
2. Season chicken breasts with salt and pepper on both sides.
3. Place chicken breasts in a baking dish.
4. In a bowl, mix together halved cherry tomatoes, chopped fresh basil, balsamic vinegar, extra virgin olive oil, minced garlic, salt, and pepper to make the relish.
5. Spoon the tomato basil relish over the chicken breasts.
6. Bake for 20-25 minutes, or until chicken is cooked through and juices run clear.
7. Serve baked chicken breasts hot, topped with tomato basil relish.

Nutrition Facts (per serving):

- Calories: 250
- Carbohydrates: 5g
- Protein: 25g
- Fat: 14g

30. Mediterranean Tuna Salad Lettuce Wraps

Prep.Time: 10 min

Cook Time: 0 min

Serving: 2

Beverage pairing: Iced Tea

Ingredients:

- 1 can (5 oz) tuna in water, drained
- 1/4 cup diced cucumber
- 1/4 cup diced red bell pepper
- 2 tablespoons diced red onion
- 2 tablespoons chopped Kalamata olives
- 2 tablespoons chopped fresh parsley
- 1 tablespoon extra virgin olive oil
- 1 tablespoon lemon juice
- Salt and pepper to taste
- Lettuce leaves for wrapping

Preparation:

1. In a bowl, combine drained tuna, diced cucumber, diced red bell pepper, diced red onion, chopped Kalamata olives, and chopped parsley.
2. Drizzle extra virgin olive oil and lemon juice over the tuna mixture. Season with salt and pepper to taste. Toss to combine.
3. Spoon the Mediterranean tuna salad onto lettuce leaves.
4. Roll up the lettuce leaves to form wraps.
5. Serve tuna salad lettuce wraps chilled or at room temperature.

Nutritional Information (per serving):

- Calories: 180
- Carbohydrates: 5g
- Protein: 20g
- Fat: 10g

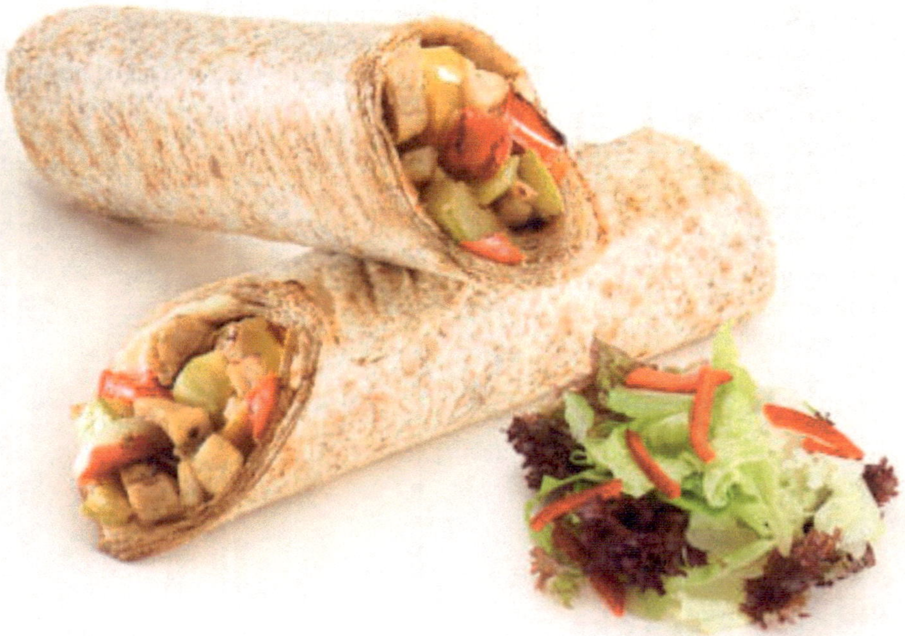

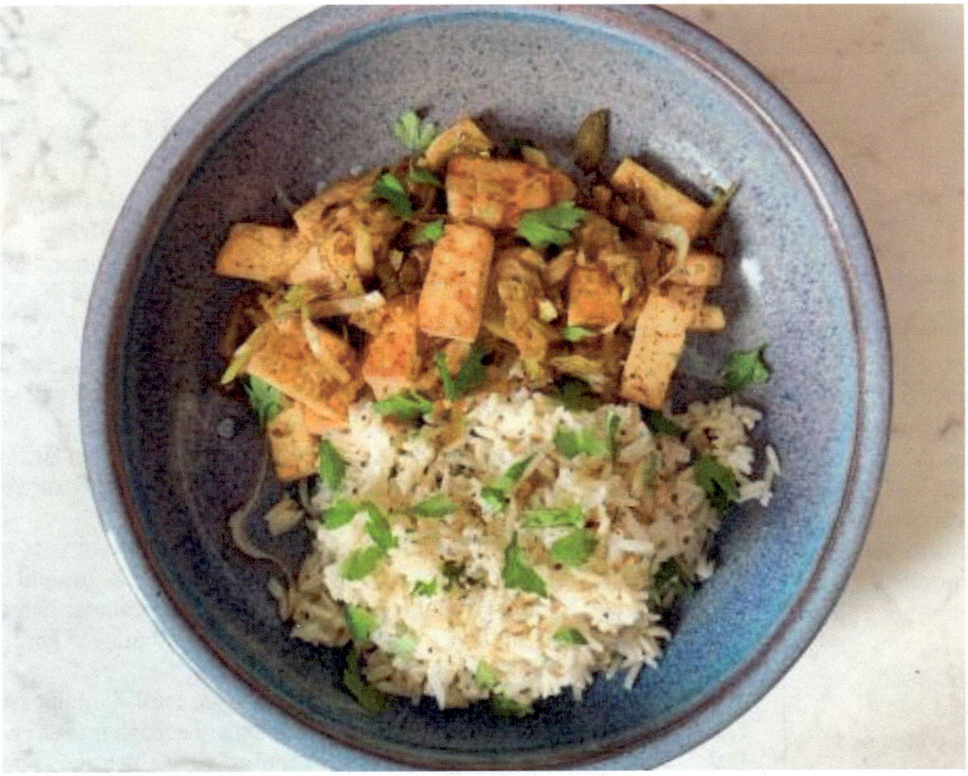

31. Vegetable and Tofu Stir-Fry with Brown Rice

Prep.Time: 15 min

Cook Time: 15 min

Serving: 2

Beverage pairing: Green Tea

Ingredients:

- 1 block (14 oz) firm tofu, pressed and cubed
- 2 cups mixed vegetables (such as bell peppers, broccoli, carrots, snap peas)
- 2 tablespoons soy sauce
- 1 tablespoon hoisin sauce
- 1 tablespoon sesame oil
- 2 cloves garlic, minced
- 1 teaspoon grated ginger
- Cooked brown rice for serving
- Sesame seeds for garnish (optional)

Preparation:

1. In a large skillet or wok, heat sesame oil over medium-high heat.
2. Add cubed tofu to the skillet and cook until golden brown on all sides. Remove tofu from the skillet and set aside.
3. In the same skillet, add minced garlic and grated ginger. Cook for 1 minute until fragrant.
4. Add mixed vegetables to the skillet and stir-fry for 3-4 minutes until tender-crisp.
5. Return cooked tofu to the skillet. Add soy sauce and hoisin sauce. Stir well to combine and coat the tofu and vegetables.
6. Cook for another 1-2 minutes until heated through.
7. Serve vegetable and tofu stir-fry over cooked brown rice.
8. Garnish with sesame seeds and chopped green onions if desired.

Nutrition Facts (per serving):

- Calories: 300
- Carbohydrates: 25g
- Protein: 20g
- Fat: 12g

32. Spaghetti Squash Primavera with Grilled Chicken

Prep.Time: 15 min

Cook Time: 30 min

Serving: 2

Beverage pairing: Lemonade

Ingredients:

- 1 medium spaghetti squash
- 2 boneless, skinless chicken breasts
- 2 cups mixed vegetables (such as bell peppers, cherry tomatoes, zucchini, mushrooms)
- 2 tablespoons olive oil
- 2 cloves garlic, minced
- 1/4 cup chopped fresh basil
- Salt and pepper to taste
- Grated Parmesan cheese for garnish (optional)

Preparation:

1. Preheat grill to medium-high heat.
2. Cut spaghetti squash in half lengthwise and scoop out the seeds.
3. Brush the cut sides of the spaghetti squash with olive oil and season with salt and pepper.
4. Place spaghetti squash halves on the grill, cut side down. Grill for 15-20 minutes, or until tender and easily pierced with a fork. Remove from heat and let cool slightly.
5. While the spaghetti squash is grilling, season chicken breasts with salt and pepper. Grill chicken breasts for 6-8 minutes per side, or until cooked through. Remove from heat and let rest for a few minutes before slicing.
6. In a skillet, heat olive oil over medium heat. Add minced garlic and cook for 1 minute until fragrant.
7. Add mixed vegetables to the skillet and sauté for 4-5 minutes until tender.
8. Use a fork to scrape the flesh of the spaghetti squash into strands.
9. Toss spaghetti squash strands with cooked vegetables and chopped fresh basil.
10. Serve spaghetti squash primavera topped with sliced grilled chicken breasts.
11. Optionally, garnish with grated Parmesan cheese before serving.

Nutritional Information (per serving):

- Calories: 350
- Carbohydrates: 20g
- Protein: 30g
- Fat: 15g

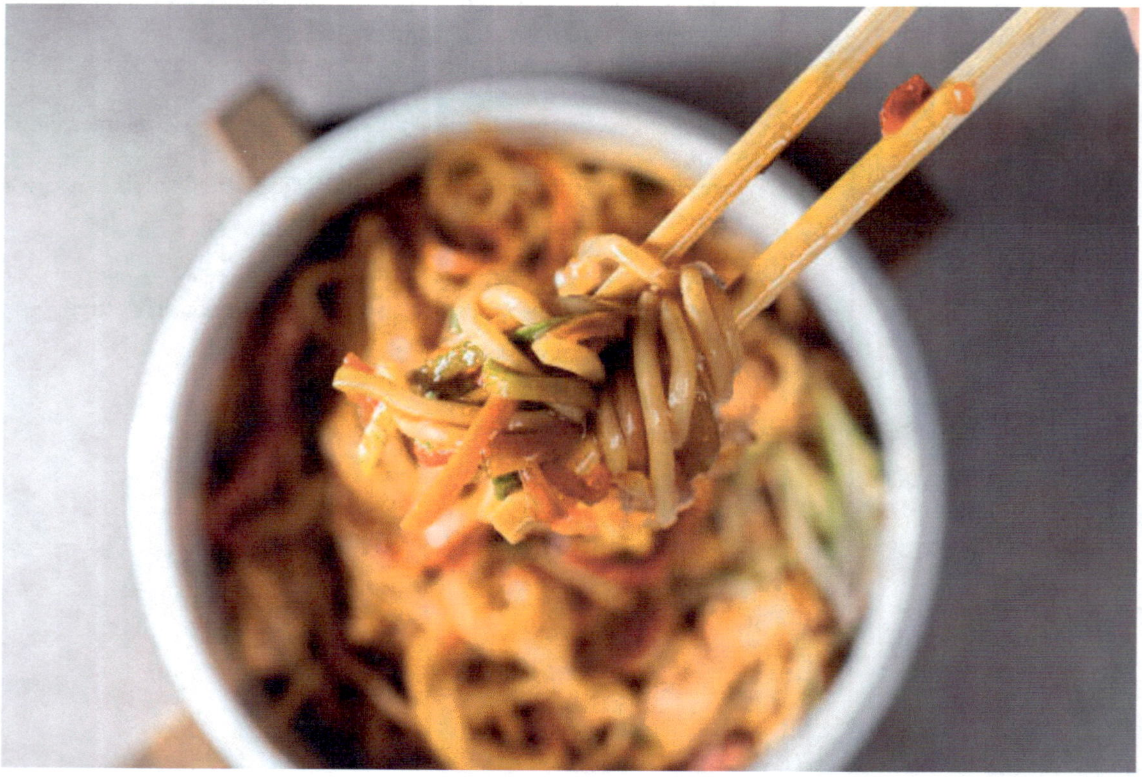

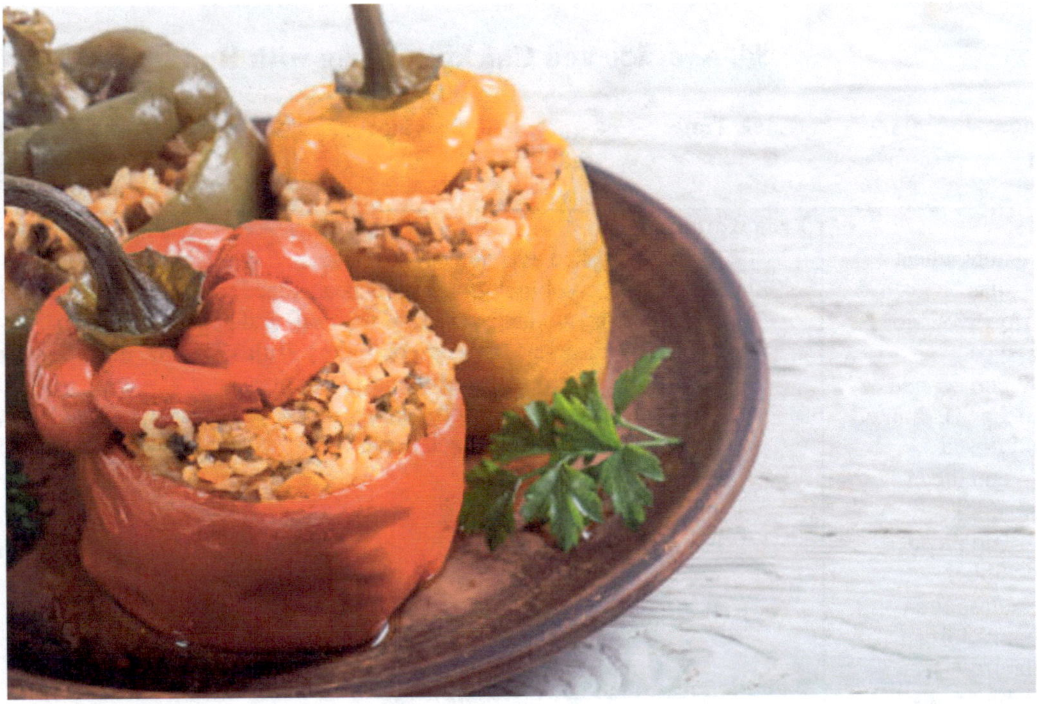

33. Turkey and Quinoa Stuffed Bell Peppers

Prep.Time: 20 min

Cook Time: 30 min

Serving: 2

Beverage pairing: Iced Tea

Ingredients:

- 2 large bell peppers, halved and seeds removed
- 1/2 cup cooked quinoa
- 1/2 lb lean ground turkey
- 1/2 cup diced tomatoes
- 1/4 cup diced onion
- 1/4 cup diced zucchini
- 1/4 cup diced mushrooms
- 1 clove garlic, minced
- 1 teaspoon Italian seasoning
- Salt and pepper to taste
- Grated mozzarella cheese for topping (optional)

Preparation:

1. Preheat oven to 375°F (190°C).
2. In a skillet, cook ground turkey over medium heat until browned.
3. Add diced onion, diced zucchini, diced mushrooms, and minced garlic to the skillet. Cook for 3-4 minutes until vegetables are softened.
4. Stir in cooked quinoa, diced tomatoes, Italian seasoning, salt, and pepper. Cook for another 2-3 minutes.
5. Place bell pepper halves in a baking dish. Spoon the turkey and quinoa mixture evenly into each pepper half.
6. Cover the dish with aluminum foil and bake for 25-30 minutes, until peppers are tender.
7. Optionally, sprinkle grated mozzarella cheese over the stuffed peppers before serving.

Nutrition Facts (per serving):

- Calories: 280
- Carbohydrates: 25g
- Protein: 20g
- Fat: 10g

34. Avocado and Chickpea Wrap with Hummus

Prep.Time: 10 min

Cook Time: 0 min

Serving: 2

Beverage pairing: Iced Tea

Ingredients:

- 2 whole wheat tortillas
- 1 ripe avocado, mashed
- 1/2 cup canned chickpeas, drained and rinsed
- 1/4 cup diced tomatoes
- 1/4 cup diced cucumber
- 2 tablespoons chopped fresh cilantro
- 2 tablespoons hummus
- Salt and pepper to taste

Preparation:

1. Spread mashed avocado evenly onto each whole wheat tortilla.
2. In a bowl, combine canned chickpeas, diced tomatoes, diced cucumber, and chopped fresh cilantro. Season with salt and pepper to taste.
3. Spoon the chickpea mixture onto the tortillas over the mashed avocado.
4. Drizzle hummus over the chickpea mixture.
5. Roll up the tortillas to form wraps.
6. Slice each wrap in half and serve.

Nutritional Information (per serving):

- Calories: 300
- Carbohydrates: 30g
- Protein: 10g
- Fat: 15g

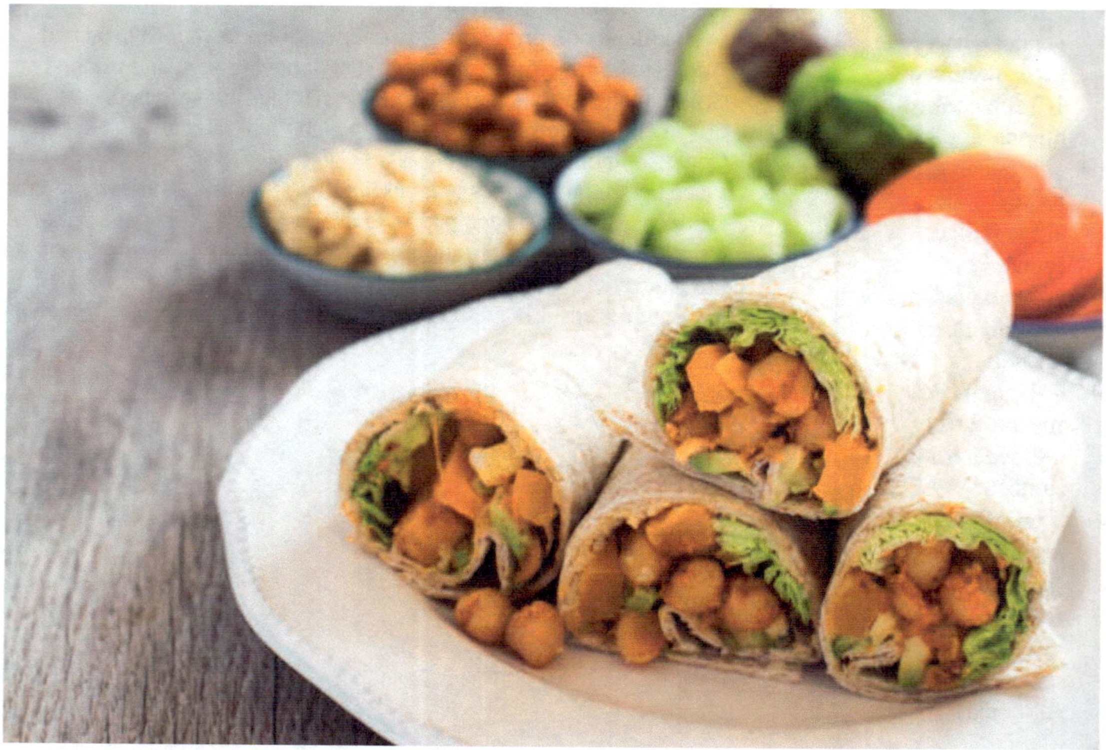

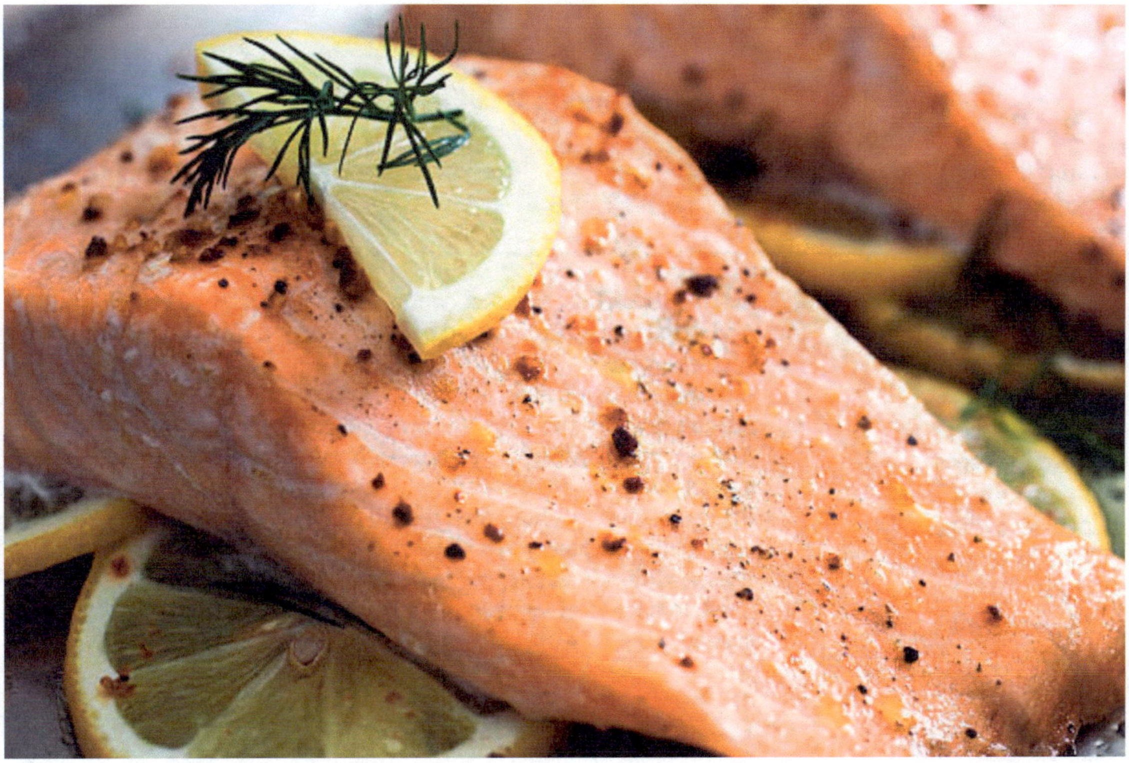

35. Baked Salmon with Dijon Mustard Glaze

Prep.Time: 5 min

Cook Time: 15 min

Serving: 2

Beverage pairing: Iced Tea

Ingredients:

- 2 salmon fillets (about 6 oz each)
- 2 tablespoons Dijon mustard
- 1 tablespoon honey
- 1 tablespoon olive oil
- 1 clove garlic, minced
- Salt and pepper to taste
- Lemon wedges for serving

Preparation:

1. Preheat oven to 400°F (200°C).
2. In a small bowl, whisk together Dijon mustard, honey, olive oil, minced garlic, salt, and pepper to make the glaze.
3. Place salmon fillets on a baking sheet lined with parchment paper.
4. Brush the Dijon mustard glaze over the salmon fillets, covering them evenly.
5. Bake salmon for 12-15 minutes, or until cooked through and flakes easily with a fork.
6. Remove from oven and let rest for a few minutes before serving.
7. Serve baked salmon hot with lemon wedges on the side.

Nutrition Facts (per serving):

- Calories: 350
- Carbohydrates: 5g
- Protein: 30g
- Fat: 20g

36. Tomato Basil Lentil Soup

Prep.Time: 10 min

Cook Time: 30 min

Serving: 4

Beverage pairing: Iced Tea

Ingredients:

- 1 cup dry green lentils, rinsed
- 4 cups vegetable broth
- 1 can (14.5 oz) diced tomatoes
- 1 onion, diced
- 2 carrots, diced
- 2 stalks celery, diced
- 2 cloves garlic, minced
- 2 tablespoons tomato paste
- 1 tablespoon olive oil
- 1 teaspoon dried basil
- Salt and pepper to taste
- Fresh basil leaves for garnish (optional)

Preparation:

1. In a large pot, heat olive oil over medium heat.
2. Add diced onion, carrots, and celery to the pot. Cook for 5-6 minutes until vegetables are softened.
3. Add minced garlic and cook for 1 minute until fragrant.
4. Stir in dried basil and tomato paste. Cook for another 1-2 minutes.
5. Add dry green lentils, vegetable broth, and diced tomatoes (with juices) to the pot.
6. Bring the soup to a boil, then reduce heat and simmer for 20-25 minutes, or until lentils are tender.
7. Season with salt and pepper to taste.
8. Serve tomato basil lentil soup hot, garnished with fresh basil leaves if desired.

Nutritional Information (per serving):

- Calories: 250
- Carbohydrates: 35g
- Protein: 15g
- Fat: 5g

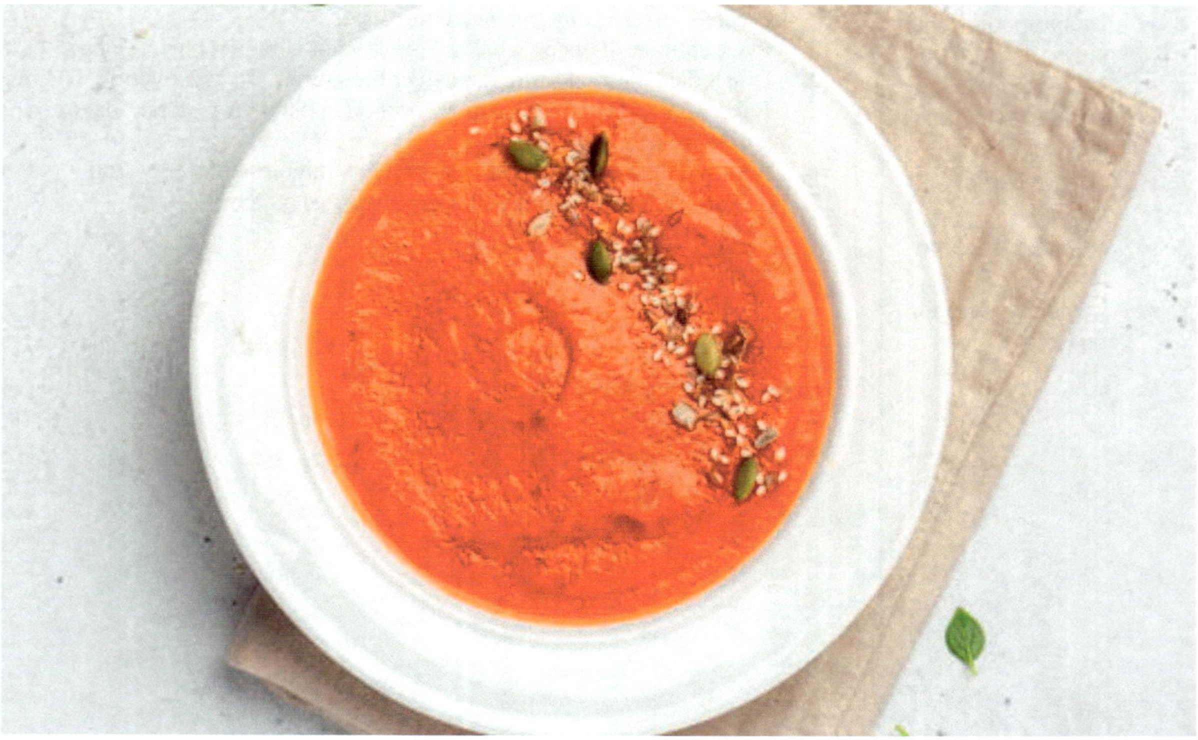

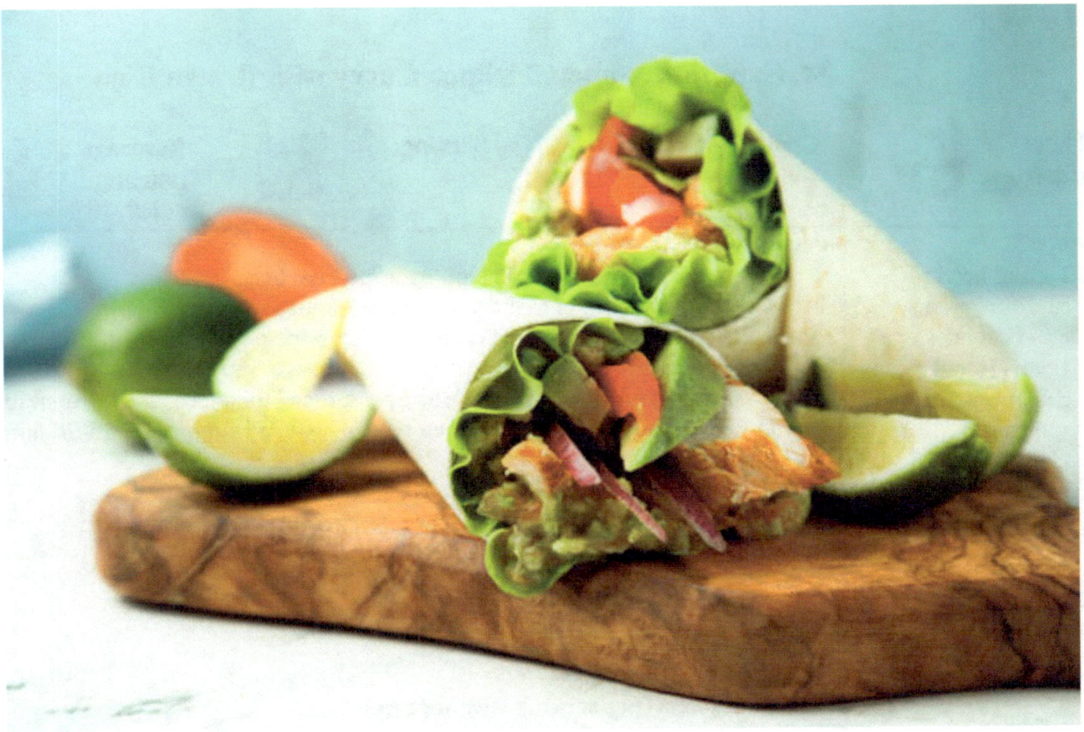

37. Chicken and Vegetable Lettuce Wraps

Prep.Time: 15 min

Cook Time: 15 min

Serving: 4

Beverage pairing: Iced Tea

Ingredients:

- 1 lb boneless, skinless chicken breasts, diced
- 2 cups mixed vegetables (such as bell peppers, water chestnuts, mushrooms, carrots)
- 1/4 cup hoisin sauce
- 2 tablespoons soy sauce
- 1 tablespoon sesame oil
- 2 cloves garlic, minced
- 1 teaspoon grated ginger
- Butter lettuce leaves for wrapping
- Chopped green onions for garnish (optional)

Preparation:

1. In a large skillet, heat sesame oil over medium-high heat.
2. Add diced chicken breasts to the skillet and cook until browned and cooked through.
3. Add mixed vegetables to the skillet and stir-fry for 3-4 minutes until tender-crisp.
4. In a small bowl, whisk together hoisin sauce, soy sauce, minced garlic, and grated ginger.
5. Pour the sauce over the chicken and vegetables in the skillet. Stir well to combine and coat evenly.
6. Cook for another 1-2 minutes until heated through.
7. Spoon chicken and vegetable mixture onto butter lettuce leaves.
8. Garnish with chopped green onions and sesame seeds if desired.
9. Serve lettuce wraps immediately.

Nutrition Facts (per serving):

- Calories: 250
- Carbohydrates: 15g
- Protein: 25g
- Fat: 10g

38. Cauliflower and Chickpea Curry with Brown Rice

Prep.Time: 15 min

Cook Time: 20 min

Serving: 4

Beverage pairing: Chai

Ingredients:

- 1 small head cauliflower, cut into florets
- 1 can (15 oz) chickpeas, drained and rinsed
- 1 onion, diced
- 2 cloves garlic, minced
- 1 can (14.5 oz) diced tomatoes
- 1 can (13.5 oz) coconut milk
- 2 tablespoons curry powder
- 1 tablespoon olive oil
- Cooked brown rice for serving
- Chopped fresh cilantro for garnish (optional)

Preparation:

1. In a large pot, heat olive oil over medium heat.
2. Add diced onion to the pot and cook until softened.
3. Add minced garlic and curry powder to the pot. Cook for 1 minute until fragrant.
4. Stir in cauliflower florets, chickpeas, diced tomatoes, and coconut milk.
5. Bring the curry to a boil, then reduce heat and simmer for 15-20 minutes, until cauliflower is tender.
6. Season with salt to taste.
7. Serve cauliflower and chickpea curry over cooked brown rice.
8. Garnish with chopped fresh cilantro if desired.

Nutrition Facts (per serving without rice):

- Calories: 280
- Carbohydrates: 20g
- Protein: 10g
- Fat: 15g

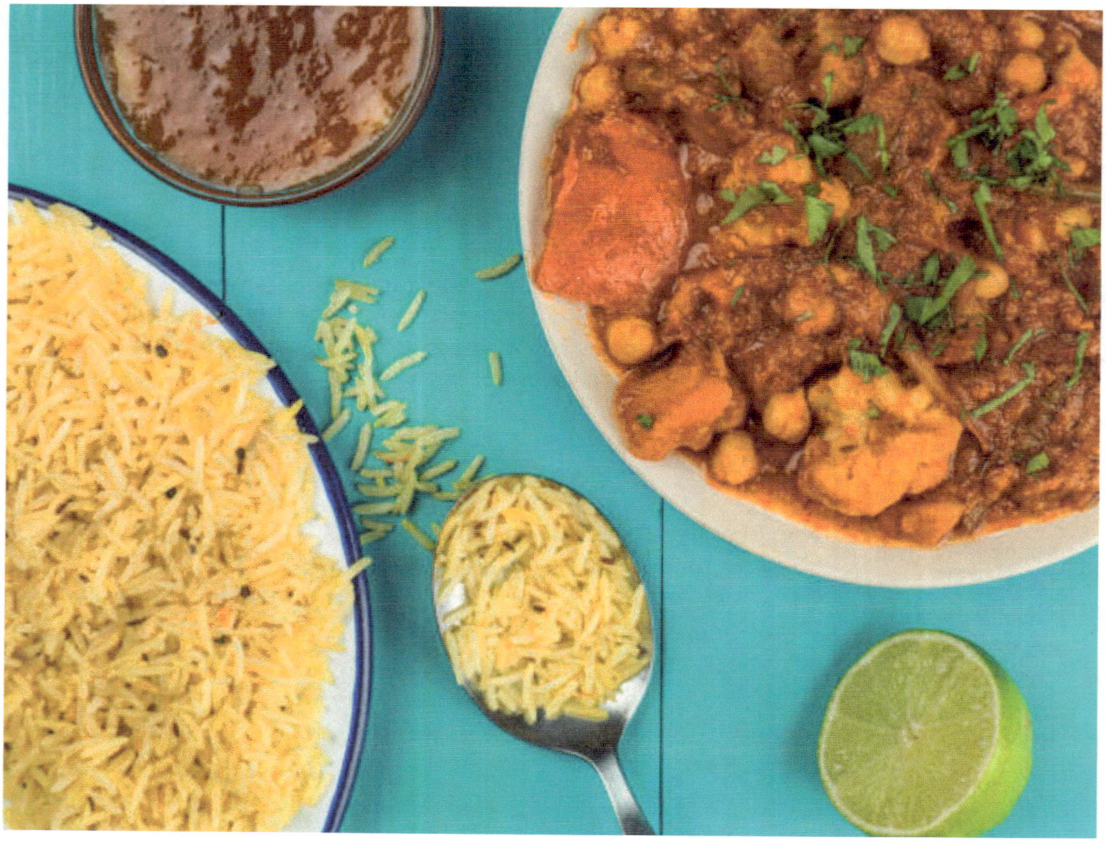

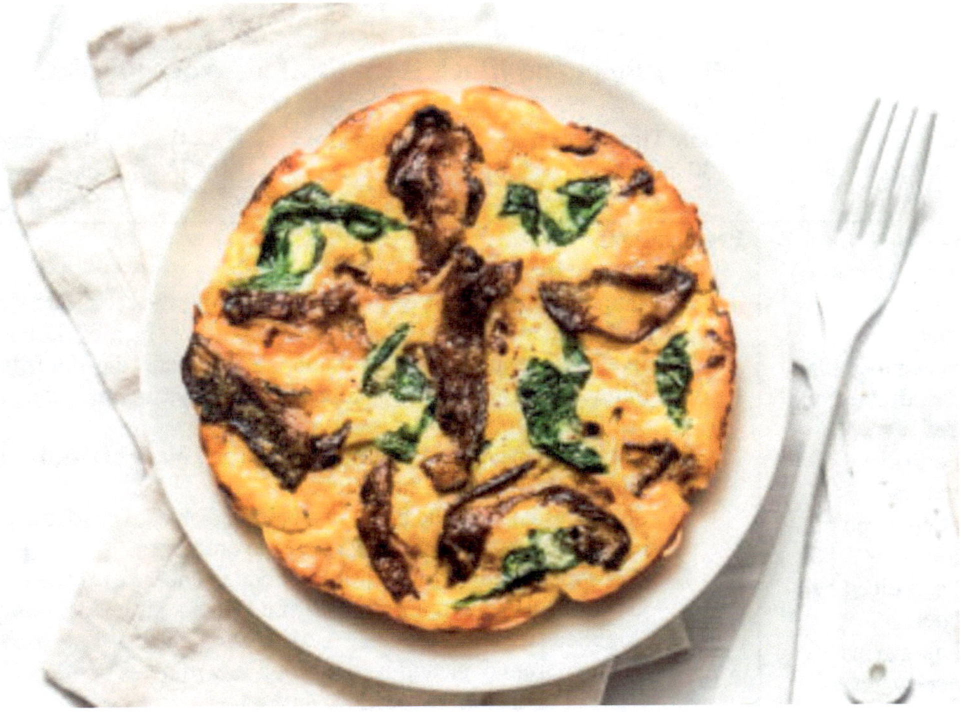

39. Spinach and Mushroom Quiche with Almond Flour Crust

Prep.Time: 20 min

Cook Time: 45 min

Serving: 6

Beverage pairing: Orange Juice

Ingredients:

- 1 1/2 cups almond flour
- 1/4 cup coconut oil, melted
- 1 tablespoon water
- 1/4 teaspoon salt
- 4 large eggs
- 1 cup almond milk (or any milk of your choice)
- 2 cups fresh spinach, chopped
- 1 cup sliced mushrooms
- 1/2 cup shredded cheese (such as cheddar or Swiss)
- 1/4 cup diced onion
- 2 cloves garlic, minced

Preparation:

1. Preheat oven to 350°F (175°C).
2. In a mixing bowl, combine almond flour, melted coconut oil, water, and salt. Mix until a dough forms.
3. Press the dough evenly into the bottom and up the sides of a 9-inch pie dish.
4. Bake the crust in the preheated oven for 10-12 minutes, until lightly golden. Remove from oven and set aside. In a skillet, heat olive oil over medium heat. Add diced onion and minced garlic to the skillet. Cook until softened and fragrant. Add sliced mushrooms to the skillet and cook until they release their moisture and start to brown.
5. Stir in chopped spinach and cook until wilted. Remove from heat and let cool slightly. In a separate bowl, whisk together eggs, almond milk, salt, and pepper. Spread the cooked vegetable mixture evenly over the baked almond flour crust. Pour the egg mixture over the vegetables in the pie dish. Sprinkle shredded cheese over the top.
6. Bake the quiche in the preheated oven for 30-35 minutes, or until the center is set and the top is golden brown. Remove from oven and let cool for a few minutes before slicing.
7. Serve spinach and mushroom quiche warm or at room temperature.

Nutrition Facts (per serving):

- Calories: 250
- Carbohydrates: 7g
- Protein: 10g
- Fat: 20g

40. Quinoa and Black Bean Stuffed Avocado Boats

Prep.Time: 15 min

Cook Time: 30 min

Serving: 4

Beverage pairing: Herbal Tea

Ingredients:

- 2 large Avocado
- 1 cup cooked quinoa
- 1 cup canned black beans, drained and rinsed
- 1/2 cup diced tomatoes
- 1/4 cup diced red onion
- 1/4 cup diced bell pepper
- 2 tablespoons chopped fresh cilantro
- 1 tablespoon lime juice
- 1 teaspoon ground cumin
- Salt and pepper to taste
- Shredded cheese for topping (optional)
- Sliced avocado for garnish (optional)

Preparation:

1. Preheat oven to 375°F (190°C).
2. Cut Avocado in half lengthwise. Scoop out the seeds and flesh to create a hollow space for the filling, leaving about 1/4 inch of flesh along the edges.
3. In a bowl, combine cooked quinoa, black beans, diced tomatoes, diced red onion, diced bell pepper, chopped fresh cilantro, lime juice, ground cumin, salt, and pepper.
4. Fill each avocado half with the quinoa and black bean mixture, pressing down lightly to pack the filling.
5. Place stuffed avocado boats in a baking dish. Cover with aluminum foil and bake for 25-30 minutes, until avacado are tender.
6. If desired, remove foil, sprinkle shredded cheese over the top of each avocado boat, and return to the oven for an additional 5 minutes until cheese is melted and bubbly.
7. Remove from oven and let cool for a few minutes before serving.
8. Garnish with sliced avocado if desired.

Nutrition Facts (per serving):

- Calories: 250
- Carbohydrates: 35g
- Protein: 10g
- Fat: 8g

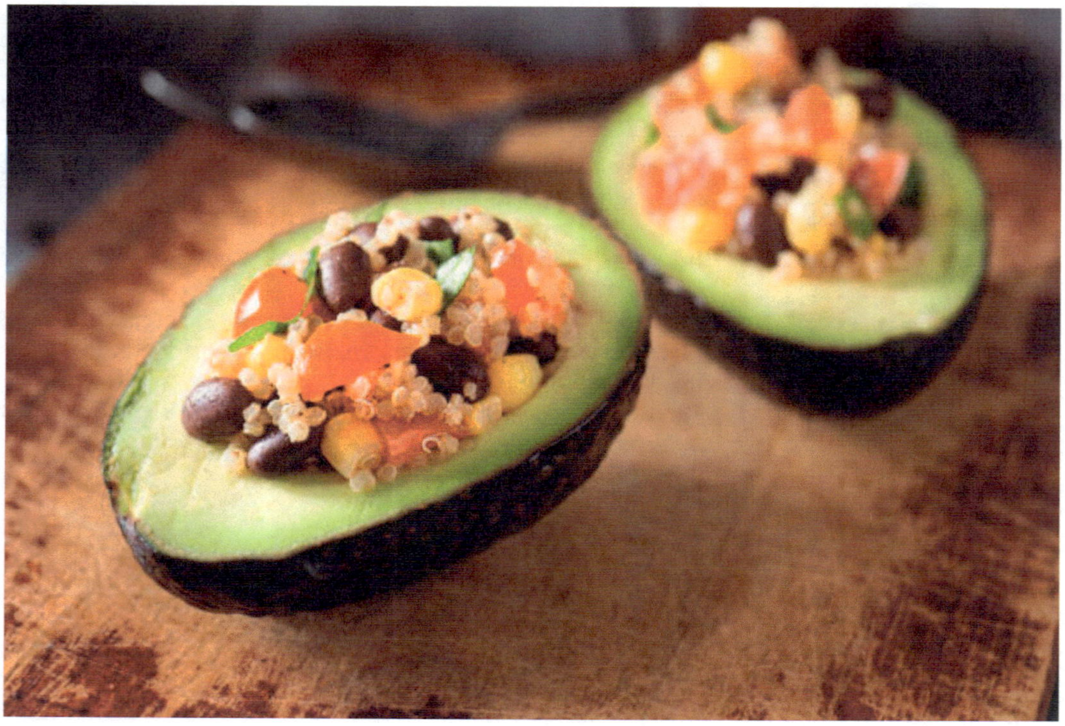

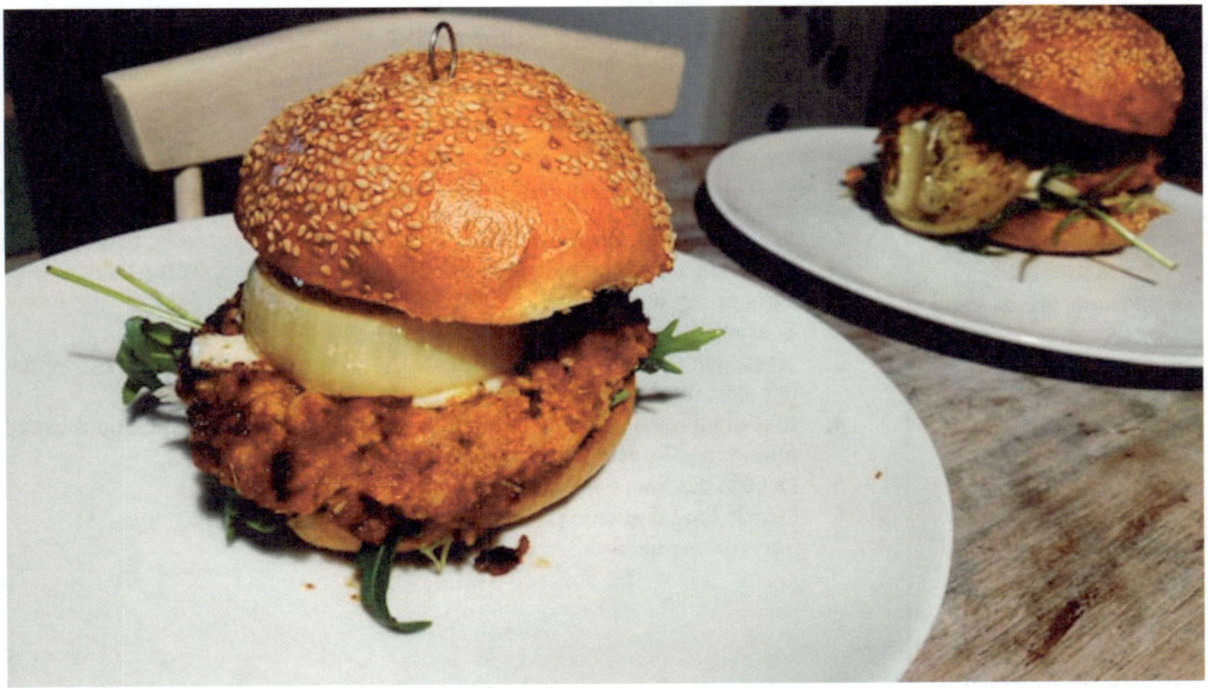

41. Lemon Herb Grilled Turkey Burgers

Prep.Time: 15 min

Cook Time: 12 min

Serving: 4

Beverage pairing: Iced Tea

Ingredients:

- 1 lb ground turkey
- 1/4 cup breadcrumbs
- 2 tablespoons chopped fresh parsley
- 1 tablespoon chopped fresh basil
- 1 tablespoon chopped fresh oregano
- 1 teaspoon lemon zest
- 1 tablespoon lemon juice
- 1 clove garlic, minced
- Salt and pepper to taste
- Whole wheat burger buns
- Lettuce leaves, tomato slices

Preparation:

1. In a large bowl, combine ground turkey, breadcrumbs, chopped parsley, basil, oregano, lemon zest, lemon juice, minced garlic, salt, and pepper. Mix until well combined.
2. Divide the turkey mixture into equal portions and shape into burger patties.
3. Preheat grill to medium-high heat.
4. Grill turkey burgers for 5-6 minutes on each side, or until cooked through and no longer pink in the center.
5. Toast whole wheat burger buns on the grill for a minute or two.
6. Assemble turkey burgers on the toasted buns with lettuce leaves, tomato slices, and other toppings of your choice.
7. Serve hot.

Nutrition Facts (per serving without bun and toppings):

- Calories: 200
- Carbohydrates: 4g
- Protein: 25g
- Fat: 9g

42. Shrimp and Avocado Salad with Lime Vinaigrette

Prep.Time: 15 min

Cook Time: 6 min

Serving: 4

Beverage pairing: Lemonade

Ingredients:

- 1 lb shrimp, peeled and deveined
- 4 cups mixed salad greens
- 1 avocado, diced
- 1/2 cup cherry tomatoes, halved
- 1/4 cup sliced red onion
- 1/4 cup sliced cucumber
- 2 tablespoons chopped fresh cilantro
- 3 tablespoons olive oil
- 2 tablespoons fresh lime juice
- 1 teaspoon honey
- 1 teaspoon Dijon mustard
- 1 clove garlic, minced

Preparation:

1. In a large bowl, combine mixed salad greens, diced avocado, halved cherry tomatoes, sliced red onion, sliced cucumber, and chopped fresh cilantro. Toss gently to combine.
2. Season shrimp with salt and pepper.
3. Heat a skillet over medium-high heat. Add shrimp and cook for 2-3 minutes per side, until pink and cooked through.
4. In a small bowl, whisk together olive oil, lime juice, honey, Dijon mustard, minced garlic, salt, and pepper to make the lime vinaigrette.
5. Drizzle the lime vinaigrette over the salad and toss to coat.
6. Divide the salad onto plates and top with cooked shrimp.
7. Serve immediately.

Nutrition Facts (per serving):

- Calories: 300
- Carbohydrates: 10g
- Protein: 25g
- Fat: 18g

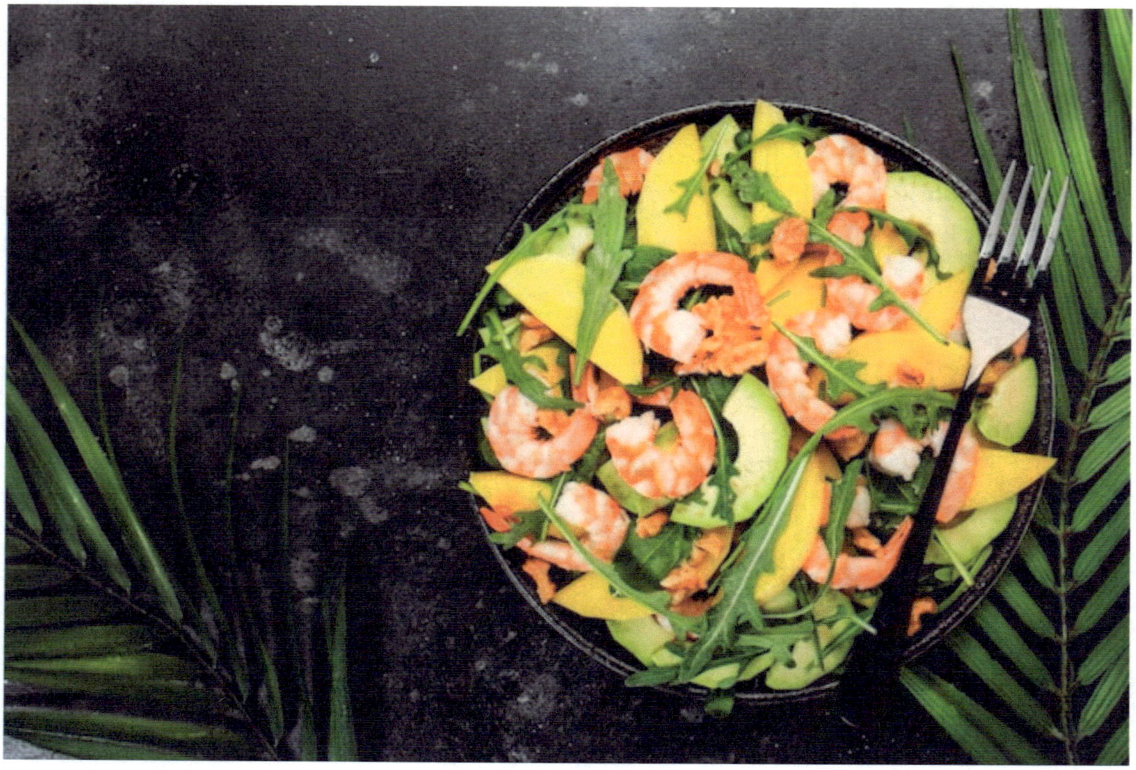

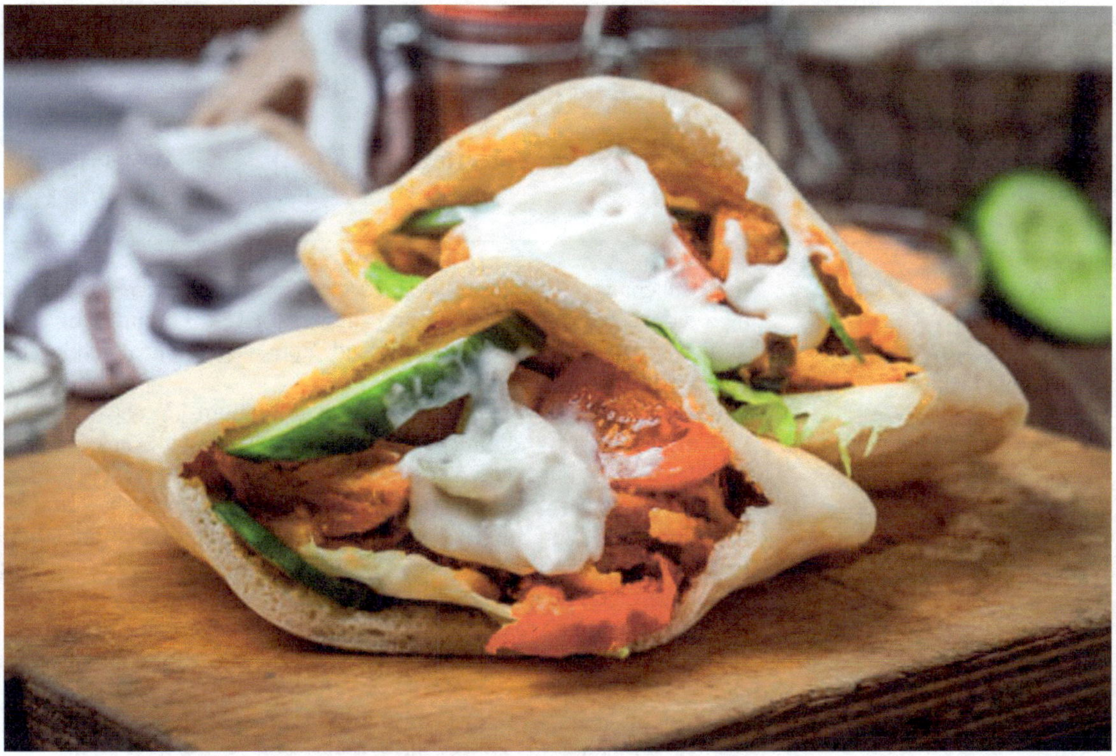

43. Greek Yogurt Chicken Pita Pocket

Prep.Time: 10 min

Cook Time: 0 min

Serving: 4

Beverage pairing: Lemonade

Ingredients:

- 2 boneless, skinless chicken breasts, cooked and sliced
- 4 whole wheat pita pockets
- 1 cup Greek yogurt
- 1 cucumber, thinly sliced
- 1/2 cup cherry tomatoes, halved
- 1/4 cup sliced red onion
- 2 tablespoons chopped fresh dill
- Salt and pepper to taste
- Lemon wedges for serving

Preparation:

1. Cut the whole wheat pita pockets in half to form pockets.
2. In a bowl, mix together Greek yogurt, chopped fresh dill, salt, and pepper.
3. Spread Greek yogurt mixture inside each pita pocket.
4. Fill each pita pocket with sliced cooked chicken breast, cucumber slices, cherry tomato halves, and sliced red onion.
5. Serve chicken pita pockets with lemon wedges on the side.

Nutrition Facts (per serving):

- Calories: 300
- Carbohydrates: 30g
- Protein: 25g
- Fat: 8g

44. Quinoa and Vegetable Stir-Fry

Prep.Time: 15 min

Cook Time: 25 min

Serving: 4

Beverage pairing: Green Tea

Ingredients:

- 1 cup quinoa, rinsed
- 2 cups water or vegetable broth
- 2 tablespoons olive oil
- 2 cloves garlic, minced
- 1 onion, thinly sliced
- 2 carrots, julienned
- 1 bell pepper, thinly sliced
- 1 cup snap peas
- 1 cup broccoli florets
- 1/4 cup soy sauce
- 1 tablespoon sesame oil
- 1 tablespoon rice vinegar
- 1 teaspoon grated ginger

Preparation:

1. In a saucepan, combine quinoa and water or vegetable broth. Bring to a boil, then reduce heat to low, cover, and simmer for 15-20 minutes, or until quinoa is cooked and water is absorbed. Remove from heat and let it sit, covered, for 5 minutes. Fluff with a fork.
2. In a large skillet or wok, heat olive oil over medium-high heat.
3. Add minced garlic and thinly sliced onion to the skillet. Cook for 2-3 minutes until onion is softened.
4. Add julienned carrots, thinly sliced bell pepper, snap peas, and broccoli florets to the skillet. Stir-fry for 4-5 minutes until vegetables are tender-crisp.
5. In a small bowl, whisk together soy sauce, sesame oil, rice vinegar, grated ginger, salt, and pepper.
6. Add cooked quinoa to the skillet with the stir-fried vegetables. Pour the soy sauce mixture over the quinoa and vegetables. Stir well to combine and coat evenly.
7. Cook for another 2-3 minutes until heated through.
8. Garnish with chopped green onions and sesame seeds if desired.
9. Serve hot.

Nutrition Facts (per serving):

- Calories: 300
- Carbohydrates: 45g
- Protein: 10g
- Fat: 10g

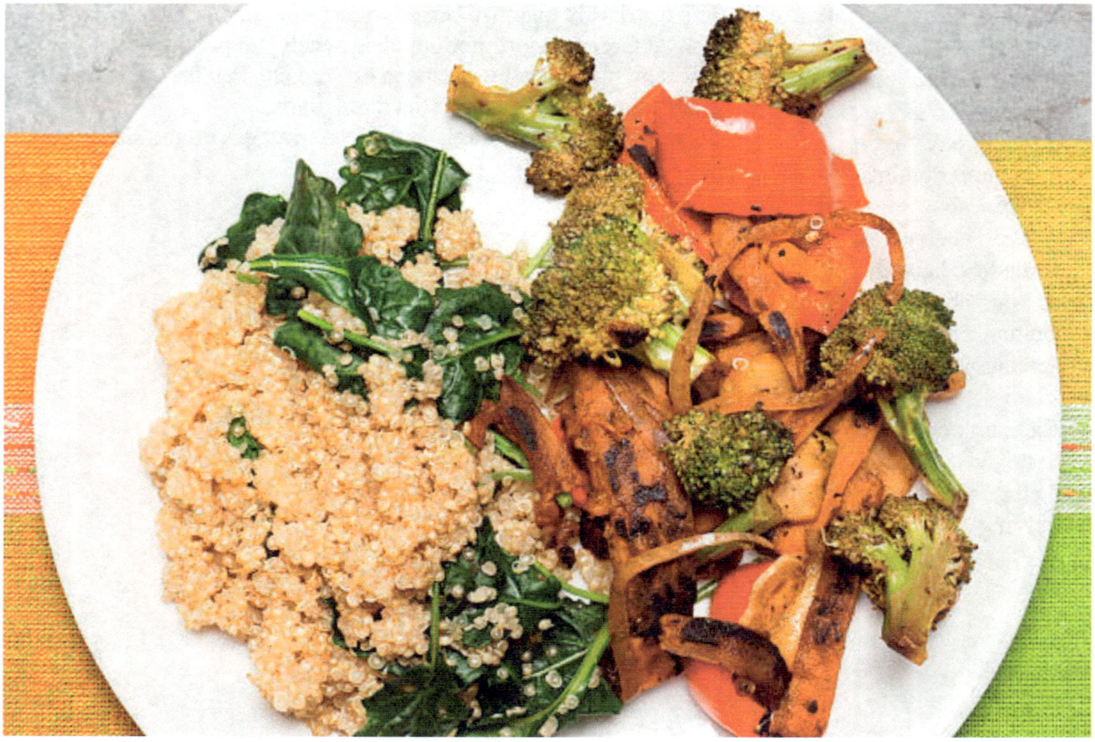

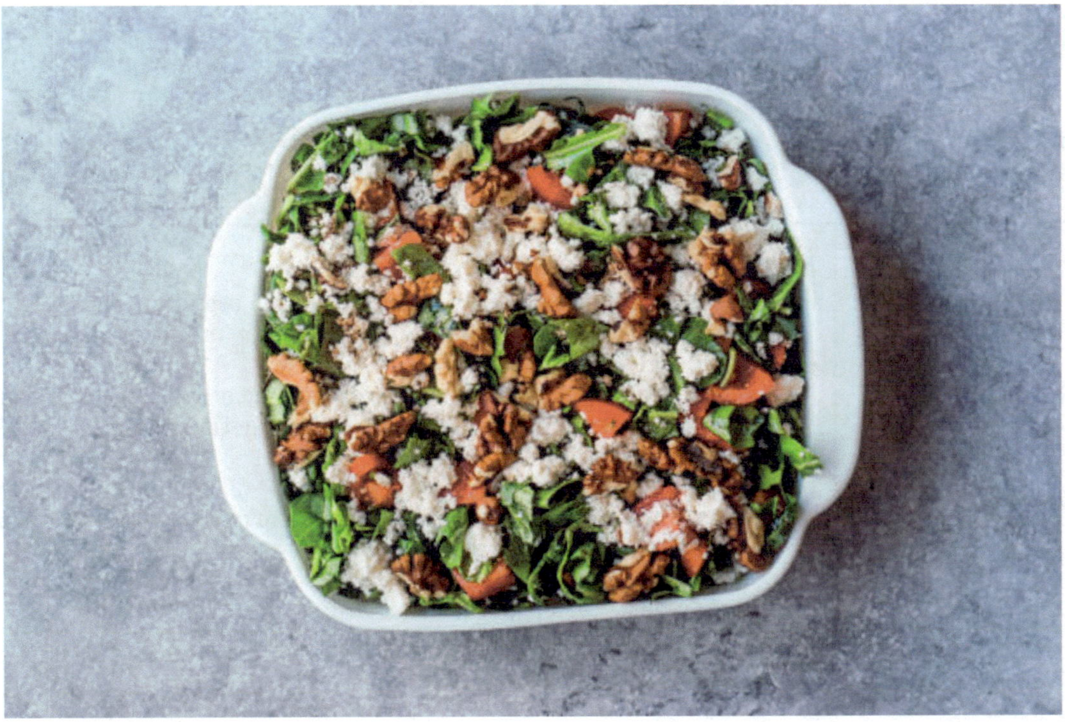

45. Turkey and Cranberry Quinoa Bowl

Prep.Time: 10 min

Cook Time: 25 min

Serving: 4

Beverage pairing: Cranberry Juice

Ingredients:

- 1 cup quinoa, rinsed
- 2 cups water or vegetable broth
- 1 lb ground turkey
- 1/2 cup dried cranberries
- 1/4 cup chopped pecans
- 1/4 cup chopped fresh parsley
- 2 tablespoons olive oil
- 1 tablespoon balsamic vinegar
- Salt and pepper to taste

Preparation:

1. In a saucepan, combine quinoa and water or vegetable broth. Bring to a boil, then reduce heat to low, cover, and simmer for 15-20 minutes, or until quinoa is cooked and water is absorbed. Remove from heat and let it sit, covered, for 5 minutes. Fluff with a fork.
2. In a skillet, heat olive oil over medium-high heat.
3. Add ground turkey to the skillet and cook until browned and cooked through.
4. Stir in cooked quinoa, dried cranberries, chopped pecans, chopped fresh parsley, and balsamic vinegar.
5. Season with salt and pepper to taste.
6. Cook for another 2-3 minutes until heated through.
7. Serve turkey and cranberry quinoa bowls hot.

Nutrition Facts (per serving):

- Calories: 350
- Carbohydrates: 30g
- Protein: 25g
- Fat: 15g

46. Baked Cod with Mediterranean Salsa

Prep.Time: 10 min

Cook Time: 15 min

Serving: 4

Beverage pairing: Lemonasde

Ingredients:

- 4 cod fillets (about 6 oz each)
- 2 tablespoons olive oil
- 2 cloves garlic, minced
- 1/2 cup diced tomatoes
- 1/4 cup diced red onion
- 1/4 cup chopped Kalamata olives
- 2 tablespoons chopped fresh parsley
- 1 tablespoon lemon juice
- 1 teaspoon dried oregano
- Salt and pepper to taste
- Lemon wedges for serving

Preparation:

1. Preheat oven to 400°F (200°C).
2. Place cod fillets on a baking sheet lined with parchment paper.
3. Drizzle olive oil over the cod fillets. Season with minced garlic, salt, and pepper.
4. In a bowl, combine diced tomatoes, diced red onion, chopped Kalamata olives, chopped fresh parsley, lemon juice, and dried oregano to make the Mediterranean salsa.
5. Spoon the Mediterranean salsa over the cod fillets, dividing it evenly.
6. Bake cod in the preheated oven for 12-15 minutes, or until fish is opaque and flakes easily with a fork.
7. Remove from oven and let rest for a few minutes before serving.
8. Serve baked cod hot with lemon wedges on the side.

Nutrition Facts (per serving):

- Calories: 250
- Carbohydrates: 5g
- Protein: 30g
- Fat: 12g

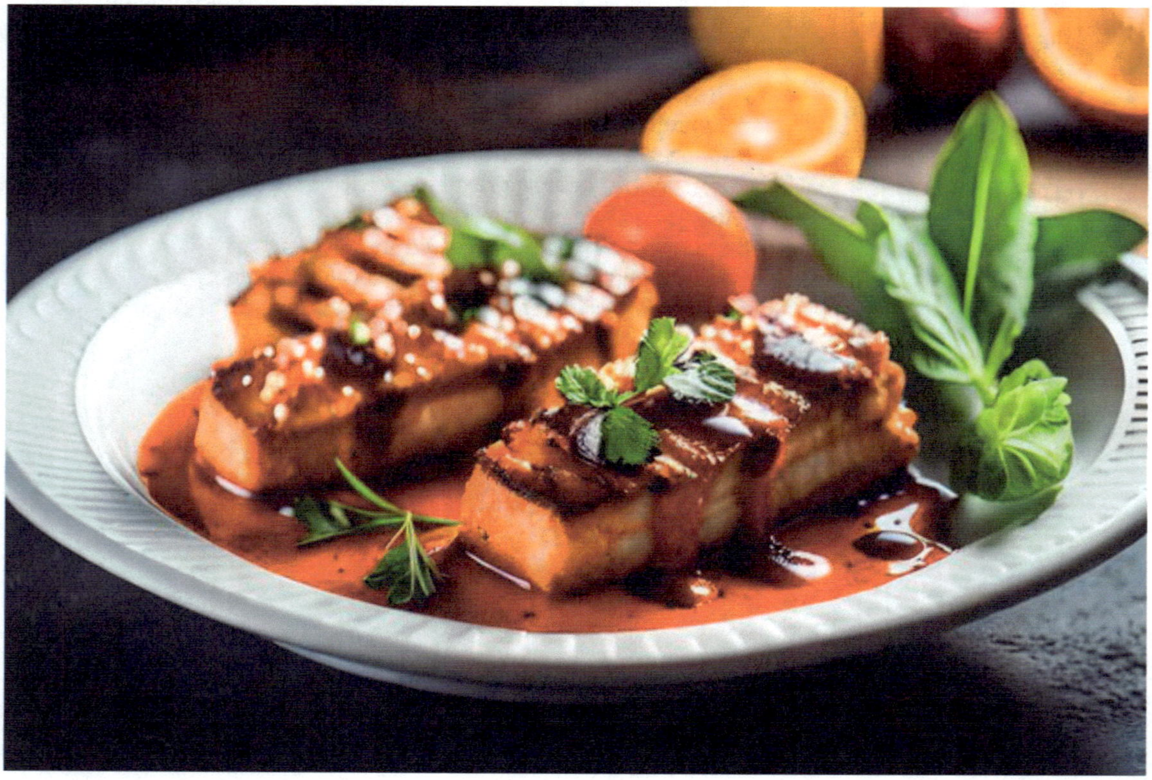

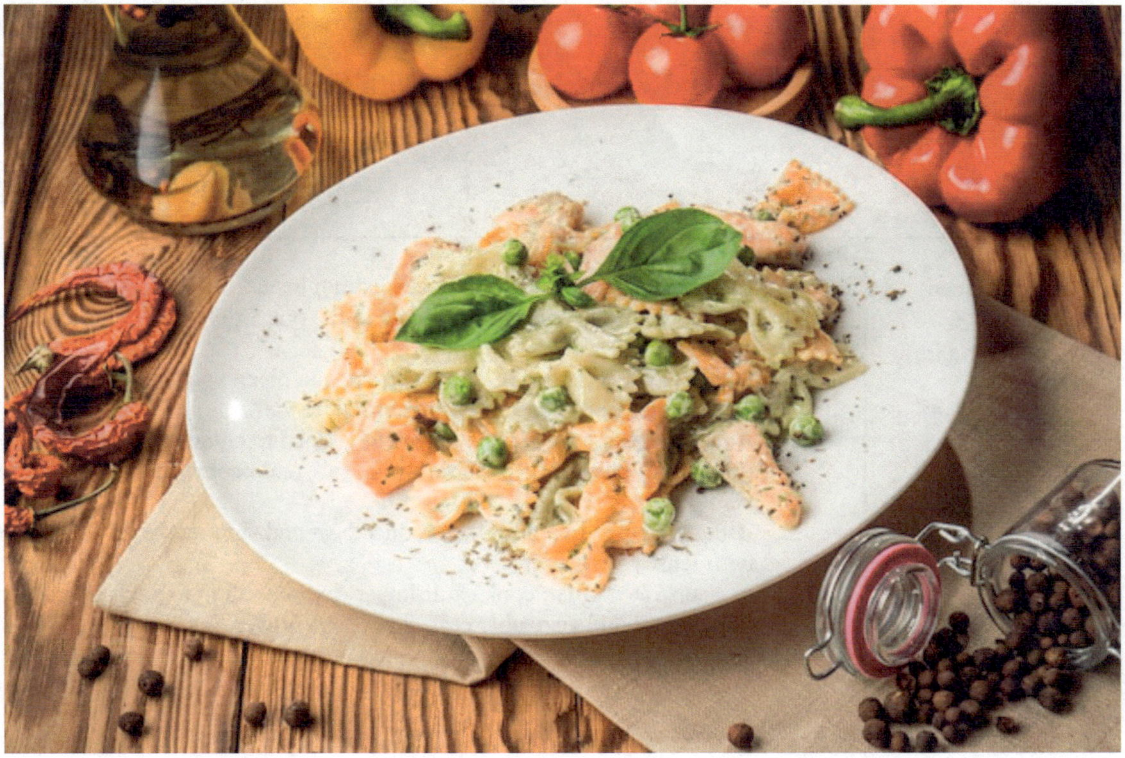

47. Caprese Zoodle Salad with Grilled Chicken

Prep.Time: 15 min

Cook Time: 16 min

Serving: 2

Beverage pairing: Lemonade

Ingredients:

- 2 medium zucchinis, spiralized into noodles
- 2 boneless, skinless chicken breasts
- 1 cup cherry tomatoes, halved
- 1 cup fresh mozzarella balls, halved
- 1/4 cup chopped fresh basil
- 2 tablespoons balsamic vinegar
- 2 tablespoons olive oil
- Salt and pepper to taste

Preparation:

1. Preheat grill to medium-high heat.
2. Season chicken breasts with salt and pepper on both sides.
3. Grill chicken breasts for 6-8 minutes per side, or until cooked through. Remove from heat and let rest for a few minutes before slicing.
4. In a large bowl, combine zucchini noodles, halved cherry tomatoes, halved fresh mozzarella balls, and chopped fresh basil.
5. In a small bowl, whisk together balsamic vinegar, olive oil, salt, and pepper to make the dressing.
6. Pour the dressing over the zucchini noodle salad and toss to coat evenly.
7. Divide the salad onto plates and top with sliced grilled chicken breasts.
8. Serve immediately.

Nutrition Facts (per serving):

- Calories: 300
- Carbohydrates: 10g
- Protein: 30g
- Fat: 15g

48. Lentil and Vegetable Curry with Cauliflower Rice

Prep.Time: 10 min

Cook Time: 35 min

Serving: 4

Beverage pairing: Mint Water

Ingredients:

- 1 cup dry green lentils, rinsed
- 4 cups vegetable broth
- 1 tablespoon olive oil
- 1 onion, diced
- 2 cloves garlic, minced
- 1 bell pepper, diced
- 2 carrots, diced
- 1 zucchini, diced
- 1 cup cauliflower rice
- 1 can (14.5 oz) diced tomatoes
- 1 can (13.5 oz) coconut milk
- 2 tablespoons curry powder
- 1 teaspoon ground turmeric

Preparation:

1. In a large pot, heat olive oil over medium heat.
2. Add diced onion and minced garlic to the pot. Cook for 2-3 minutes until softened.
3. Stir in diced bell pepper, diced carrots, and diced zucchini. Cook for another 3-4 minutes until vegetables are slightly tender.
4. Add dry green lentils, vegetable broth, diced tomatoes (with juices), coconut milk, curry powder, ground turmeric, salt, and pepper to the pot. Stir well to combine.
5. Bring the curry to a boil, then reduce heat and simmer for 25-30 minutes, or until lentils are tender.
6. In a separate skillet, cook cauliflower rice according to package instructions.
7. Serve lentil and vegetable curry over cauliflower rice.
8. Garnish with chopped fresh cilantro if desired.

Nutrition Facts (per serving):

- Calories: 350
- Carbohydrates: 40g
- Protein: 15g
- Fat: 15g

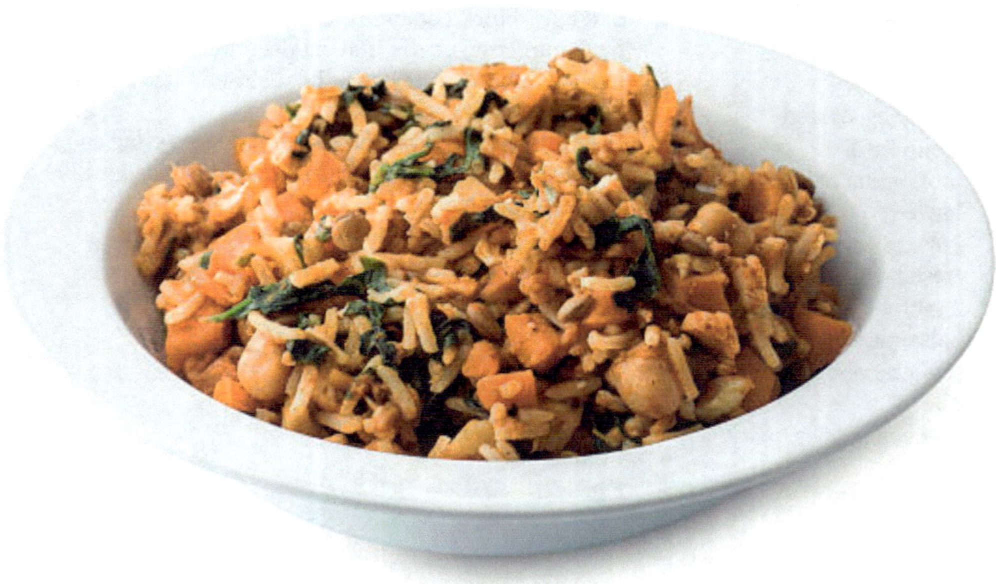

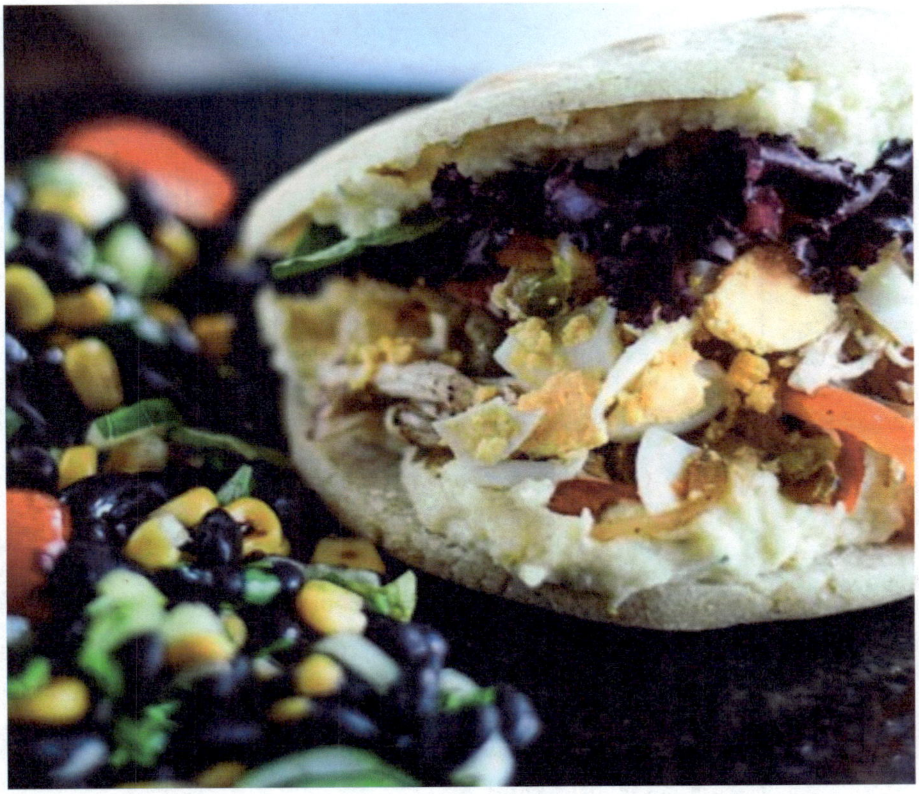

49. Chicken and Black Bean Pita Bread

Prep.Time: 10 min

Cook Time: 15 min

Serving: 4

Beverage pairing: Pineaaple Juice

Ingredients:

- 1 lb boneless, skinless chicken breasts
- 1 cup cooked brown rice
- 1 can (15 oz) black beans, drained and rinsed
- 1 cup corn kernels
- 1 bell pepper, diced
- 1/4 cup diced red onion
- 1/4 cup chopped fresh cilantro
- 1 teaspoon ground cumin
- 1 teaspoon chili powder
- Pita Bread
- 1 avocado, sliced
- Lime wedges for serving

Preparation:

1. Season chicken breasts with ground cumin, chili powder, salt, and pepper on both sides.
2. Grill or cook chicken breasts in a skillet over medium-high heat until browned and cooked through. Remove from heat and let rest for a few minutes before slicing.
3. In a large bowl, combine cooked brown rice, black beans, corn kernels, diced bell pepper, diced red onion, chopped fresh cilantro, salt, and pepper. Toss gently to combine.
4. Divide the rice and bean mixture into bowls.
5. Top each bowl with sliced grilled chicken breasts and sliced avocado.
6. Serve chicken and black bean Pita Bread with lime wedges on the side.

Nutrition Facts (per serving):

- Calories: 350
- Carbohydrates: 40g
- Protein: 30g
- Fat: 10g

50. Spinach and Feta Turkey Burgers

Prep.Time: 15 min

Cook Time: 12 min

Serving: 4

Beverage pairing: Iced Tea

Ingredients:

- 1 lb ground turkey
- 1 cup fresh spinach, chopped
- 1/4 cup crumbled feta cheese
- 2 tablespoons chopped fresh parsley
- 1 clove garlic, minced
- Salt and pepper to taste
- Whole wheat burger buns
- Lettuce leaves, tomato slices, and other toppings of your choice

Preparation:

1. In a large bowl, combine ground turkey, chopped fresh spinach, crumbled feta cheese, chopped fresh parsley, minced garlic, salt, and pepper. Mix until well combined.
2. Divide the turkey mixture into equal portions and shape into burger patties.
3. Preheat grill to medium-high heat.
4. Grill turkey burgers for 5-6 minutes on each side, or until cooked through and no longer pink in the center.
5. Toast whole wheat burger buns on the grill for a minute or two.
6. Assemble turkey burgers on the toasted buns with lettuce leaves, tomato slices, and other toppings of your choice.
7. Serve hot.

Nutrition Facts (per serving without bun and toppings):

- Calories: 250
- Carbohydrates: 2g
- Protein: 30g
- Fat: 15g

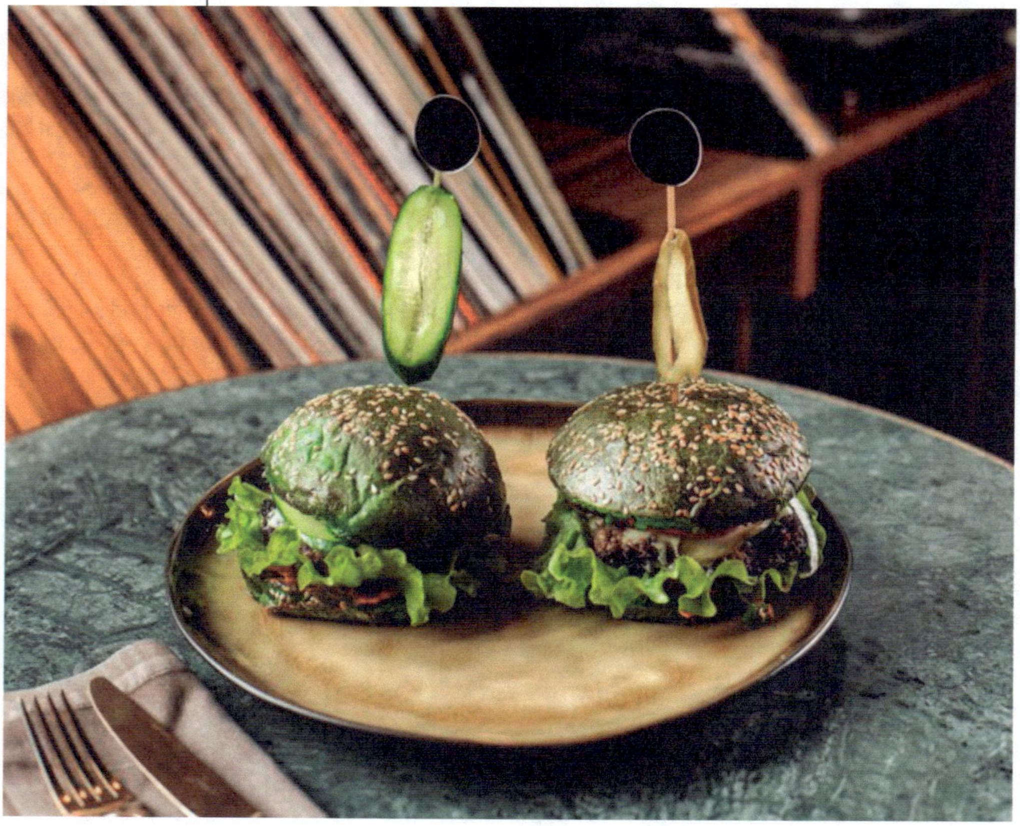

Your Kindness is Key

Share Your Experience, Share Your Strength

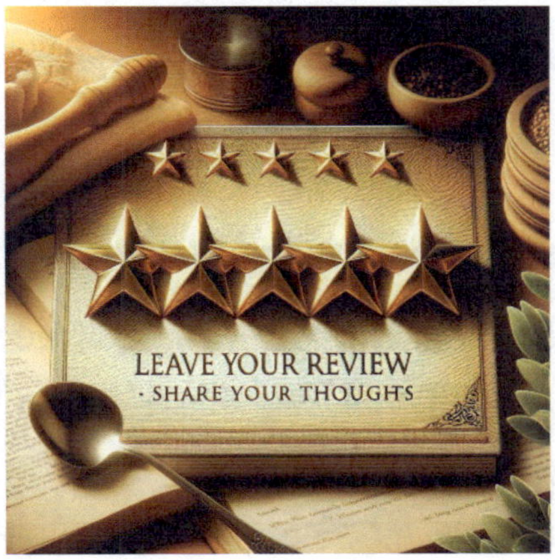

"Helping one person might not change the whole world, but it could change the world for one person." - Anonymous

---

Do you remember what it was like when you first heard the words "Type 2 Diabetes?" Perhaps it felt like a mountain you weren't sure you could climb.

Maybe it was daunting, thinking about the changes you'd have to make in your life, especially with your diet. It's a journey many embark on feeling uncertain and alone.

But you've found a companion on this journey, haven't you? Type 2 Diabetes Cookbook Beginner's Quick & Easy Recipes for Delicious Diabetes Diets by Lily Anders has been with you, offering guidance, delicious recipes, and a sense of control over your diabetes that perhaps you didn't feel before.

Imagine if you could light the path for someone just starting on this journey. Someone who feels lost in the sea of information, unsure of where to turn for reliable, practical advice on managing their diabetes through diet. Your experience, shared through a review, could be the beacon they need.

This isn't just about leaving a review; it's about extending a hand, offering support, and sharing the strength that comes from knowledge and community. Your words could help another person find their footing, making their journey a bit easier and less lonely.

So, here's my humble request on behalf of a fellow journeyer you've yet to meet:

Please take a moment to share your experience with the book. Your insights could be the very thing another person needs to hear to take that first, brave step toward a healthier, happier life with diabetes. Your review, a simple act of kindness, asks for nothing in return yet offers immeasurable value.

To leave your review, just follow this link:

https://www.amazon.com/dp/1963939352

If the thought of helping another soul on their diabetes journey warms your heart, then you're exactly who I hoped to reach with this book. Welcome to a community where kindness, support, and shared victories pave the way to a better life.

I'm beyond grateful for your help in spreading the word and even more excited to continue providing you with the knowledge and recipes to make managing diabetes not just manageable, but enjoyable.

Click the QR Code Here!

Thank you from the deepest places in my heart. Your generosity makes all the difference.

Lily Anders

P.S. - Sharing is caring, they say. If you believe this book has brought value to your life and could do the same for someone else, consider sharing it with them. It's another beautiful way to change a life, one meal at a time.

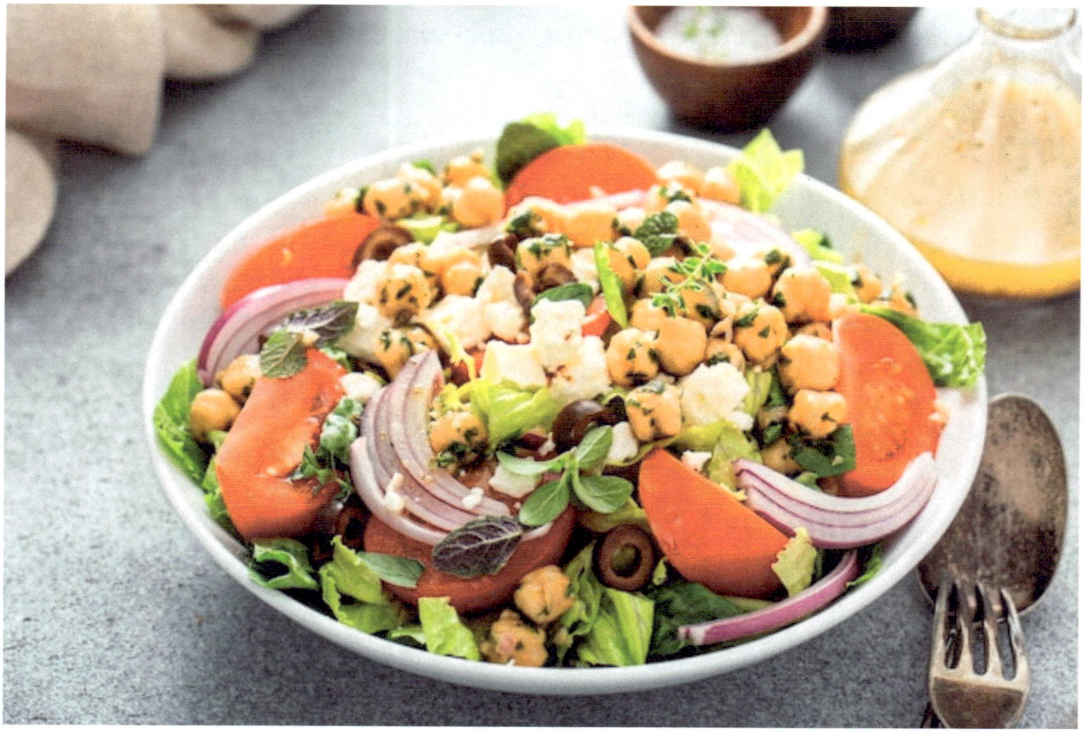

51. Quinoa and Chickpea Salad with Lemon Tahini Dressing

Prep.Time: 15 min

Cook Time: 20 min

Serving: 4

Beverage pairing: Green Tea

Ingredients:

- 1 cup quinoa, rinsed
- 2 cups water or vegetable broth
- 1 can (15 oz) chickpeas, drained and rinsed
- 1 cucumber, diced
- 1 bell pepper, diced
- 1/4 cup chopped red onion
- 1/4 cup chopped fresh parsley
- 1/4 cup chopped fresh mint
- 1/4 cup tahini
- 3 tablespoons fresh lemon juice
- 2 tablespoons water
- 1 clove garlic, minced
- 1 teaspoon honey or maple syrup

Preparation:

1. In a saucepan, combine quinoa and water or vegetable broth. Bring to a boil, then reduce heat to low, cover, and simmer for 15-20 minutes, or until quinoa is cooked and water is absorbed. Remove from heat and let it sit, covered, for 5 minutes. Fluff with a fork and let it cool.
2. In a large bowl, combine cooked quinoa, chickpeas, diced cucumber, diced bell pepper, chopped red onion, chopped fresh parsley, and chopped fresh mint. Toss gently to combine.
3. In a small bowl, whisk together tahini, fresh lemon juice, water, minced garlic, honey or maple syrup, and salt to make the lemon tahini dressing.
4. Pour the lemon tahini dressing over the quinoa and chickpea salad. Toss until everything is evenly coated.
5. Season with additional salt and pepper to taste if needed.
6. Serve quinoa and chickpea salad chilled or at room temperature.

Nutrition Facts (per serving):

- Calories: 300
- Carbohydrates: 40g
- Protein: 10g
- Fat: 12g

52. Salmon and Asparagus Foil Packets

Prep.Time: 10 min

Cook Time: 20 min

Serving: 4

Beverage pairing: Water

Ingredients:

- 4 salmon fillets
- 1 bunch asparagus, trimmed
- 2 tablespoons olive oil
- 2 cloves garlic, minced
- 1 lemon, sliced
- Salt and pepper to taste
- Fresh dill for garnish (optional)

Preparation:

1. Preheat oven to 400°F (200°C).
2. Cut four sheets of aluminum foil, large enough to wrap each salmon fillet and asparagus.
3. Place a salmon fillet on each piece of foil.
4. Arrange asparagus spears around the salmon fillets.
5. Drizzle olive oil over the salmon and asparagus.
6. Sprinkle minced garlic over the salmon and asparagus.
7. Season with salt and pepper to taste.
8. Place lemon slices on top of each salmon fillet.
9. Fold the edges of the foil to create packets, sealing tightly.
10. Place foil packets on a baking sheet.
11. Bake in the preheated oven for 15-20 minutes, or until salmon is cooked through and flakes easily with a fork.
12. Carefully open the foil packets and transfer salmon and asparagus to plates.
13. Garnish with fresh dill if desired.
14. Serve hot.

Nutrition Facts (per serving):

- Calories: 300
- Carbohydrates: 6g
- Protein: 30g
- Fat: 18g

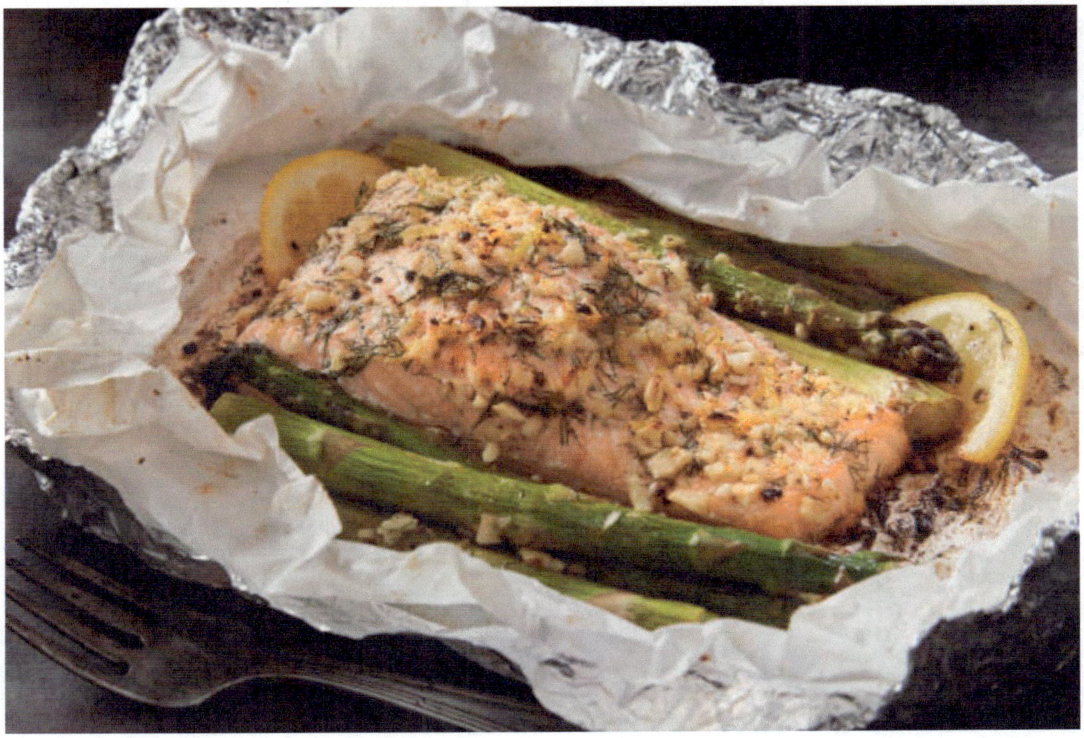

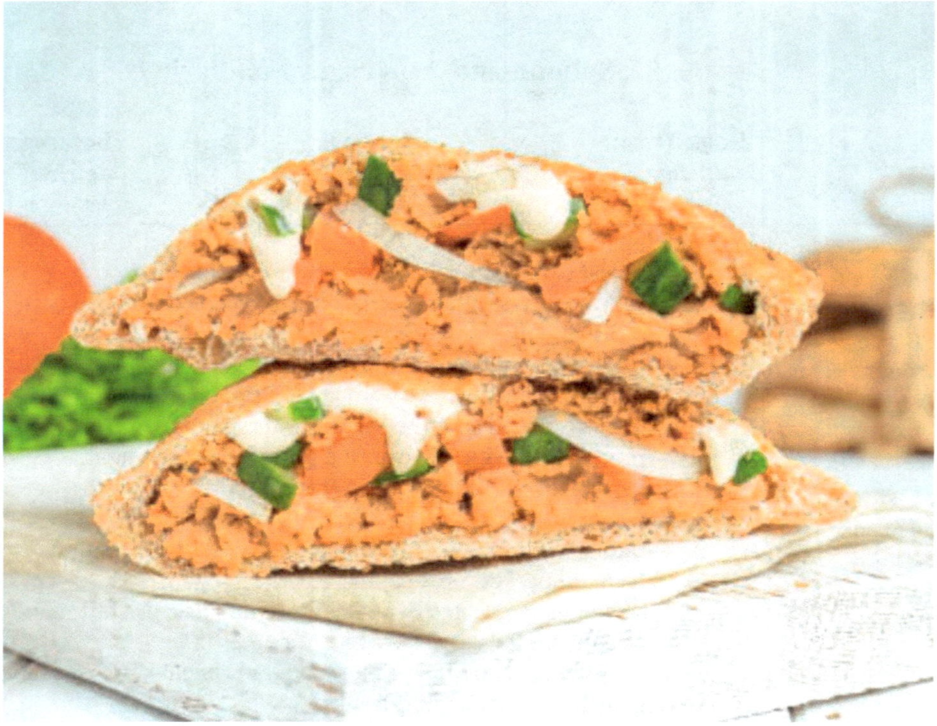

53. Roasted Vegetable and Hummus Wrap

Prep.Time: 15 min

Cook Time: 0 min

Serving: 4

Beverage pairing: Iced Tea

Ingredients:

- 4 whole wheat tortillas
- 1 cup hummus
- 2 cups mixed roasted vegetables (such as bell peppers, zucchini, eggplant, red onion)
- 1 cup fresh spinach leaves
- Salt and pepper to taste

Preparation:

1. Lay out whole wheat tortillas on a flat surface.
2. Spread 1/4 cup of hummus onto each tortilla.
3. Divide mixed roasted vegetables evenly among the tortillas.
4. Top each tortilla with fresh spinach leaves.
5. Season with salt and pepper to taste.
6. Roll up the tortillas tightly to form wraps.
7. Cut each wrap in half diagonally.
8. Serve roasted vegetable and hummus wraps immediately or wrap them tightly in foil or plastic wrap for later.

Nutrition Facts (per serving):

- Calories: 250
- Carbohydrates: 30g
- Protein: 10g
- Fat: 10g

54. Turkey and Quinoa Stuffed Acorn Squash

Prep.Time: 15 min

Cook Time: 45 min

Serving: 4

Beverage pairing: Apple Cider

Ingredients:

- 2 acorn squash, halved and seeds removed
- 1 cup quinoa, rinsed
- 2 cups vegetable broth
- 1 lb ground turkey
- 1 onion, diced
- 2 cloves garlic, minced
- 1 teaspoon dried thyme
- 1 teaspoon dried sage
- Salt and pepper to taste
- 1/2 cup dried cranberries
- 1/4 cup chopped fresh parsley

Preparation:

1. Preheat oven to 400°F (200°C).
2. Place acorn squash halves, cut side down, on a baking sheet lined with parchment paper. Bake for 30-35 minutes, or until squash is tender when pierced with a fork.
3. In a saucepan, combine quinoa and vegetable broth. Bring to a boil, then reduce heat to low, cover, and simmer for 15-20 minutes, or until quinoa is cooked and liquid is absorbed. Remove from heat and let it sit, covered, for 5 minutes. Fluff with a fork.
4. In a skillet, cook ground turkey over medium heat until browned and cooked through.
5. Add diced onion and minced garlic to the skillet with the cooked turkey. Cook for 2-3 minutes until softened.
6. Stir in dried thyme, dried sage, salt, and pepper to taste.
7. Add cooked quinoa, dried cranberries, chopped fresh parsley, and chopped pecans (if using) to the skillet with the turkey mixture. Stir to combine.
8. Fill each roasted acorn squash half with the turkey and quinoa stuffing.
9. Serve turkey and quinoa stuffed acorn squash hot.

Nutrition Facts (per serving):

- Calories: 350
- Carbohydrates: 40g
- Protein: 25g
- Fat: 12g

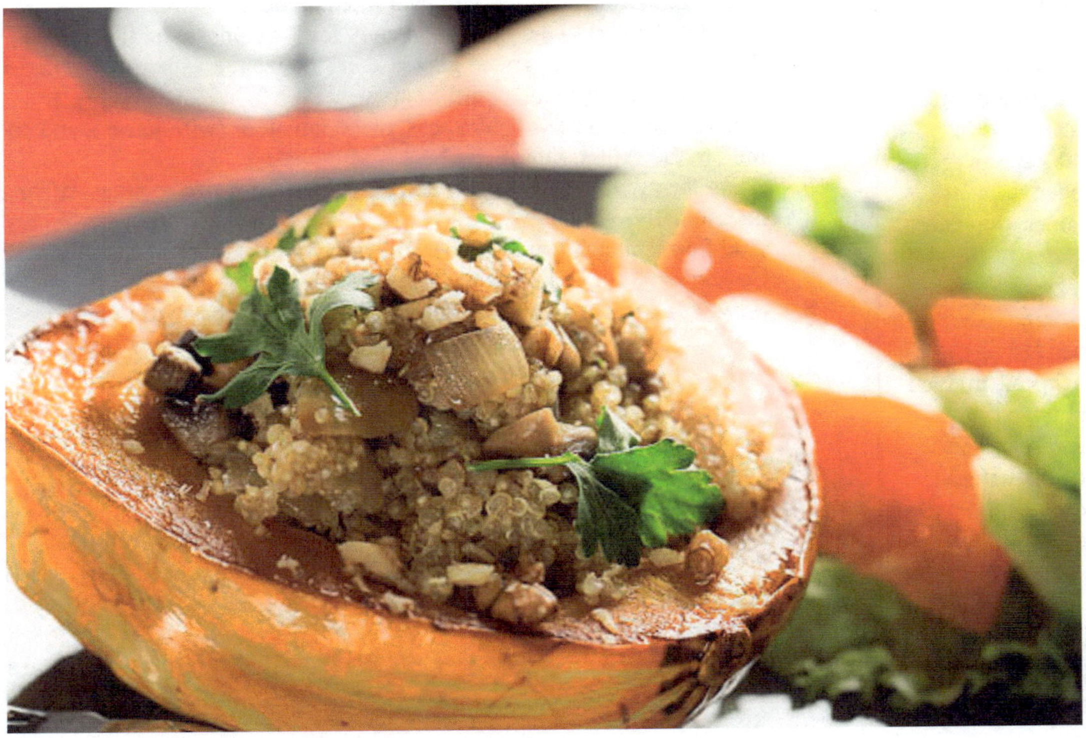

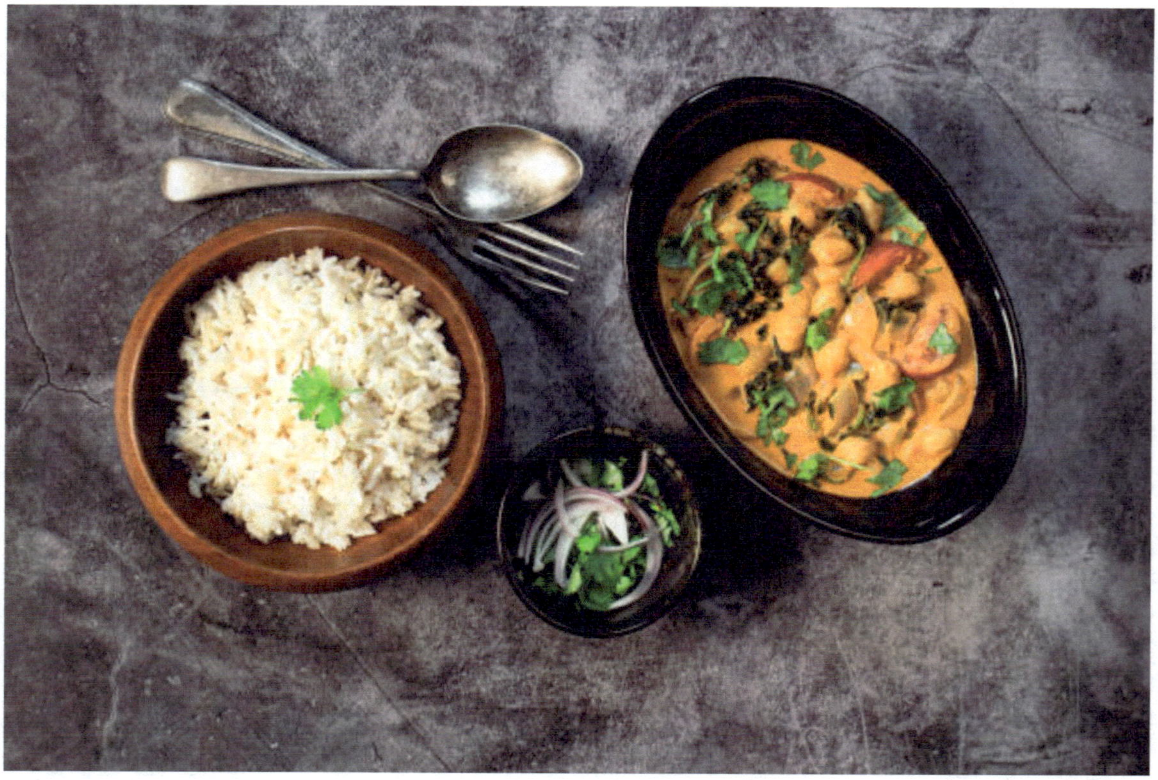

55. Chickpea and Spinach Curry with Basmati Rice

Prep.Time: 10 min

Cook Time: 20 min

Serving: 4

Beverage pairing: Coffee

Ingredients:

- 1 tablespoon olive oil
- 1 onion, diced
- 2 cloves garlic, minced
- 1 tablespoon grated ginger
- 1 tablespoon curry powder
- 1 teaspoon ground turmeric
- 1 can (15 oz) chickpeas, drained and rinsed
- 1 can (14.5 oz) diced tomatoes
- 1 can (13.5 oz) coconut milk
- 4 cups fresh spinach leaves
- Cooked basmati rice for serving

Preparation:

1. In a large skillet, heat olive oil over medium heat.
2. Add diced onion to the skillet and cook for 3-4 minutes until softened.
3. Stir in minced garlic, grated ginger, curry powder, and ground turmeric. Cook for another minute until fragrant.
4. Add drained and rinsed chickpeas, diced tomatoes (with juices), and coconut milk to the skillet. Stir to combine.
5. Bring the mixture to a simmer and let it cook for 10-15 minutes, stirring occasionally.
6. Add fresh spinach leaves to the skillet and cook until wilted.
7. Season with salt and pepper to taste.
8. Serve chickpea and spinach curry hot over cooked basmati rice.

Nutrition Facts (per serving):

- Calories: 250
- Carbohydrates: 20g
- Protein: 8g
- Fat: 15g

56. Greek Chicken and Orzo Salad

Prep.Time: 15 min

Cook Time: 15 min

Serving: 4

Beverage pairing: Lemonade

Ingredients:

- 1 lb boneless, skinless chicken breasts
- 1 tablespoon olive oil
- 2 cups cooked orzo pasta
- 1 cucumber, diced
- 1 bell pepper, diced
- 1/4 cup sliced Kalamata olives
- 1/4 cup crumbled feta cheese
- 2 tablespoons chopped fresh parsley
- 2 tablespoons chopped fresh dill
- 2 tablespoons lemon juice
- 1 tablespoon red wine vinegar
- 1 clove garlic, minced

Preparation:

1. Season chicken breasts with salt and pepper on both sides.
2. Heat olive oil in a skillet over medium-high heat.
3. Add chicken breasts to the skillet and cook for 6-7 minutes per side, or until cooked through and no longer pink in the center. Remove from heat and let rest for a few minutes before slicing.
4. In a large bowl, combine cooked orzo pasta, diced cucumber, diced bell pepper, sliced Kalamata olives, crumbled feta cheese, chopped fresh parsley, and chopped fresh dill.
5. In a small bowl, whisk together lemon juice, red wine vinegar, minced garlic, salt, and pepper to make the dressing.
6. Pour the dressing over the orzo salad and toss to coat evenly.
7. Divide the orzo salad onto plates and top with sliced grilled chicken breasts.
8. Serve Greek chicken and orzo salad immediately.

Nutrition Facts (per serving):

- Calories: 350
- Carbohydrates: 30g
- Protein: 30g
- Fat: 12g

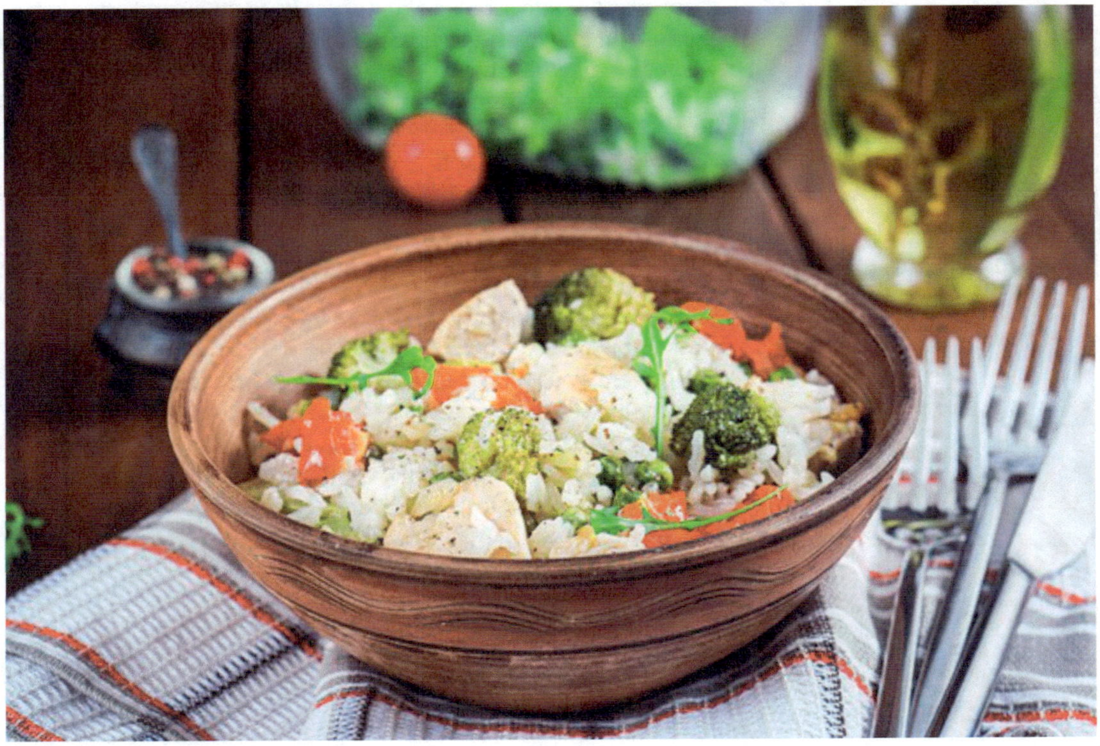

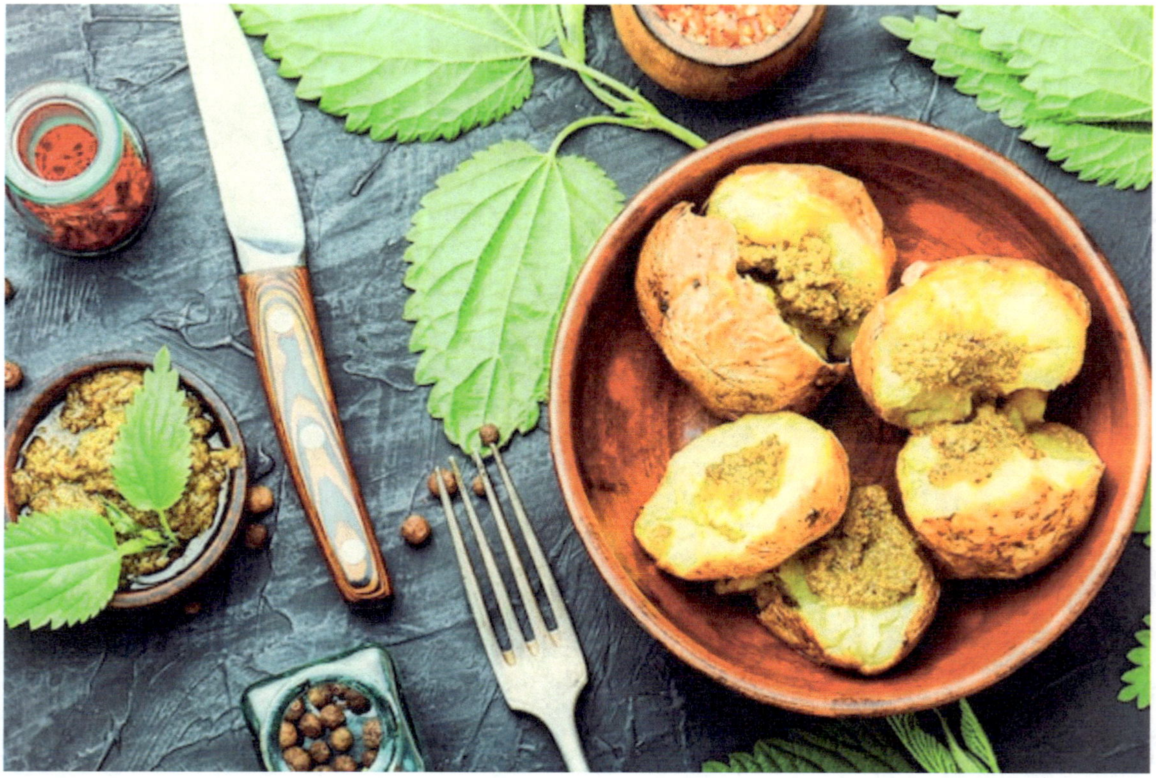

57. Broccoli and Cheddar Stuffed Sweet Potatoes

Prep.Time:	Cook Time:	Serving:	Beverage pairing:
10 min	60 min	4	Apple cider

Ingredients:

- 4 medium sweet potatoes
- 2 cups broccoli florets
- 1 tablespoon olive oil
- 1 onion, diced
- 2 cloves garlic, minced
- 1/2 cup shredded cheddar cheese
- Salt and pepper to taste

Preparation:

1. Preheat oven to 400°F (200°C).
2. Wash sweet potatoes and pierce them several times with a fork.
3. Place sweet potatoes on a baking sheet lined with parchment paper.
4. Bake sweet potatoes in the preheated oven for 45-60 minutes, or until tender when pierced with a fork.
5. In the meantime, steam or boil broccoli florets until tender. Drain and set aside.
6. Heat olive oil in a skillet over medium heat.
7. Add diced onion to the skillet and cook for 3-4 minutes until softened.
8. Stir in minced garlic and cook for another minute until fragrant.
9. Cut a slit lengthwise in each baked sweet potato and gently fluff the insides with a fork.
10. Stuff each sweet potato with cooked broccoli florets and sautéed onion and garlic mixture.
11. Top stuffed sweet potatoes with shredded cheddar cheese.
12. Return stuffed sweet potatoes to the oven and bake for an additional 5 minutes, or until cheese is melted and bubbly. Season with salt and pepper to taste. Serve broccoli and cheddar stuffed sweet potatoes hot.

Nutrition Facts (per serving):

- Calories: 250
- Carbohydrates: 40g
- Protein: 7g
- Fat: 8g

58. Turkey and Avocado Lettuce Wraps

Prep.Time: 15 min

Cook Time: 15 min

Serving: 4

Beverage pairing: Iced Tea

Ingredients:

- 1 lb ground turkey
- 1 tablespoon olive oil
- 1 onion, diced
- 2 cloves garlic, minced
- 1 teaspoon ground cumin
- 1 teaspoon chili powder
- Salt and pepper to taste
- 1 avocado, diced
- 1/4 cup diced tomatoes
- 1/4 cup chopped fresh cilantro
- Juice of 1 lime
- 8 large lettuce leaves (such as butter lettuce or romaine)

Preparation:

1. Heat olive oil in a skillet over medium heat.
2. Add diced onion and minced garlic to the skillet. Cook until softened, about 2-3 minutes.
3. Add ground turkey to the skillet. Cook, breaking up the meat with a spatula, until browned and cooked through.
4. Stir in ground cumin, chili powder, salt, and pepper. Cook for another 2-3 minutes.
5. Remove skillet from heat and stir in diced avocado, diced tomatoes, chopped fresh cilantro, and lime juice.
6. Spoon the turkey mixture onto lettuce leaves.
7. Roll up the lettuce leaves to form wraps.
8. Serve turkey and avocado lettuce wraps immediately.

Nutrition Facts (per serving, 2 wraps):

- Calories: 250
- Carbohydrates: 7g
- Protein: 25g
- Fat: 15g

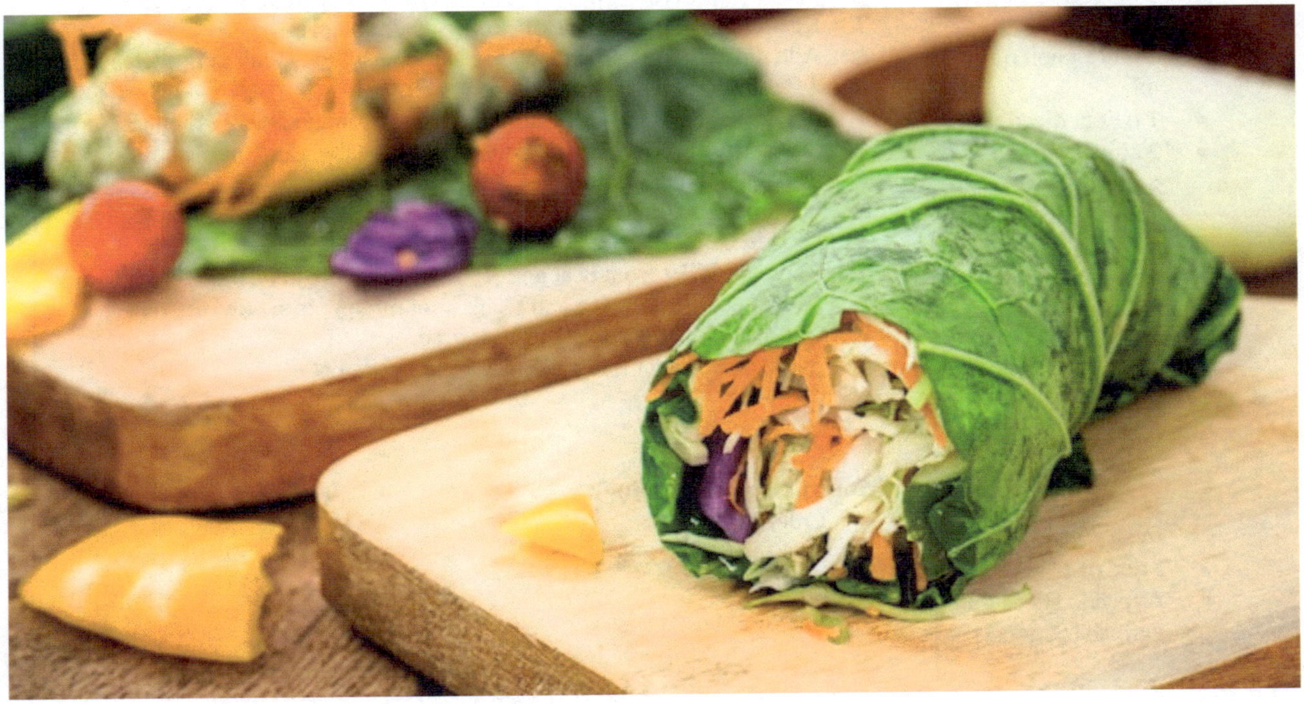

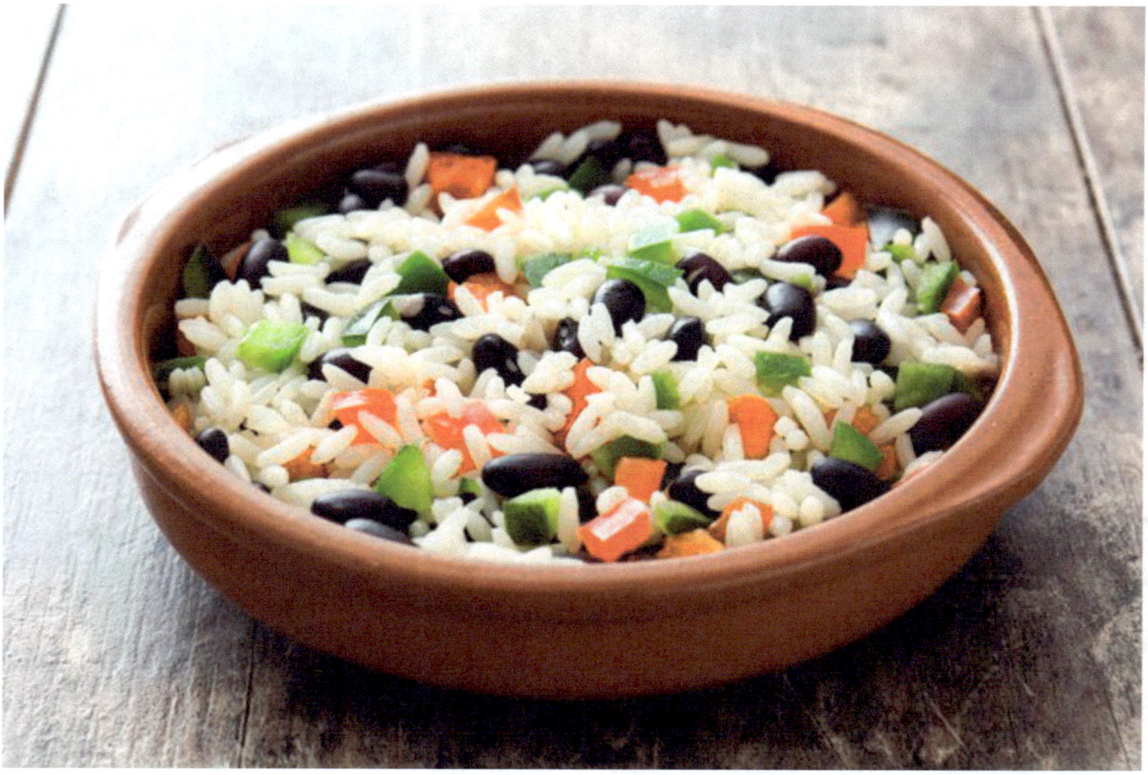

59. Cauliflower Rice and Black Bean Bowl

Prep.Time: 15 min

Cook Time: 15 min

Serving: 4

Beverage pairing: Iced Tea

Ingredients:

- 1 head cauliflower, riced
- 1 tablespoon olive oil
- 1 onion, diced
- 2 cloves garlic, minced
- 1 bell pepper, diced
- 1 cup cooked black beans
- 1 teaspoon ground cumin
- 1 teaspoon chili powder
- Salt and pepper to taste
- 1/4 cup chopped fresh cilantro
- Juice of 1 lime
- Avocado slices for garnish (optional)

Preparation:

1. In a food processor, pulse cauliflower florets until they resemble rice.
2. Heat olive oil in a large skillet over medium heat.
3. Add diced onion and minced garlic to the skillet. Cook until softened, about 2-3 minutes.
4. Add diced bell pepper to the skillet. Cook for another 2-3 minutes.
5. Stir in cauliflower rice and cooked black beans. Cook until cauliflower rice is tender, about 5-7 minutes.
6. Season with ground cumin, chili powder, salt, and pepper. Stir well to combine.
7. Remove skillet from heat and stir in chopped fresh cilantro and lime juice.
8. Divide cauliflower rice and black bean mixture into bowls.
9. Garnish with avocado slices if desired.
10. Serve cauliflower rice and black bean bowls hot.

Nutrition Facts (per serving):

- Calories: 200
- Carbohydrates: 25g
- Protein: 8g
- Fat: 8g

60. Lemon Garlic Shrimp Pasta with Zucchini Noodles

Prep.Time: 15 min

Cook Time: 10 min

Serving: 4

Beverage pairing: Lemonade

Ingredients:

- 1 lb shrimp, peeled and deveined
- 4 medium zucchinis, spiralized into noodles
- 2 tablespoons olive oil
- 4 cloves garlic, minced
- 1 teaspoon red pepper flakes
- Juice of 1 lemon
- Zest of 1 lemon
- Salt and pepper to taste
- Chopped fresh parsley for garnish
- Grated Parmesan cheese for garnish (optional)

Preparation:

1. Heat olive oil in a large skillet over medium heat.
2. Add minced garlic and red pepper flakes to the skillet. Cook until fragrant, about 1 minute.
3. Add shrimp to the skillet. Cook until shrimp turn pink and opaque, about 2-3 minutes per side.
4. Stir in spiralized zucchini noodles, lemon juice, and lemon zest. Cook for another 2-3 minutes until zucchini noodles are heated through but still slightly crisp.
5. Season with salt and pepper to taste.
6. Remove skillet from heat and garnish with chopped fresh parsley and grated Parmesan cheese if desired.
7. Serve lemon garlic shrimp pasta immediately.

Nutrition Facts (per serving):

- Calories: 250
- Carbohydrates: 10g
- Protein: 30g
- Fat: 10g

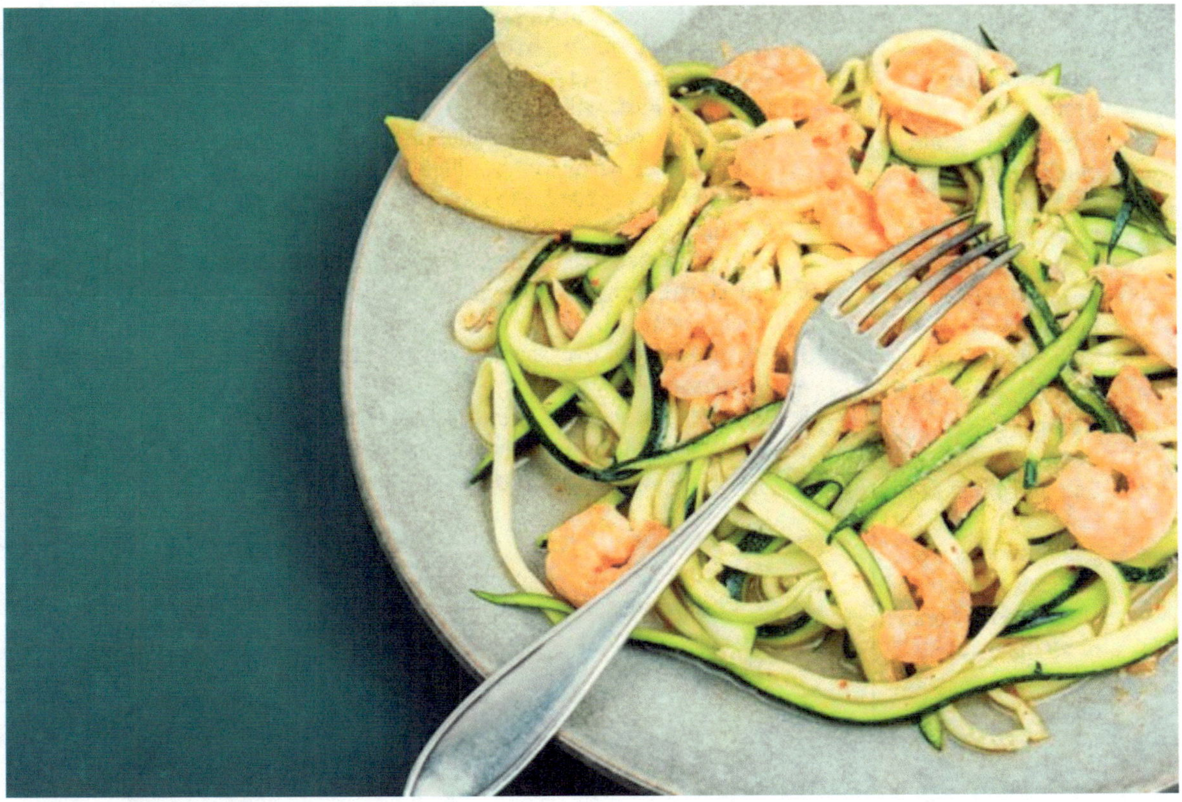

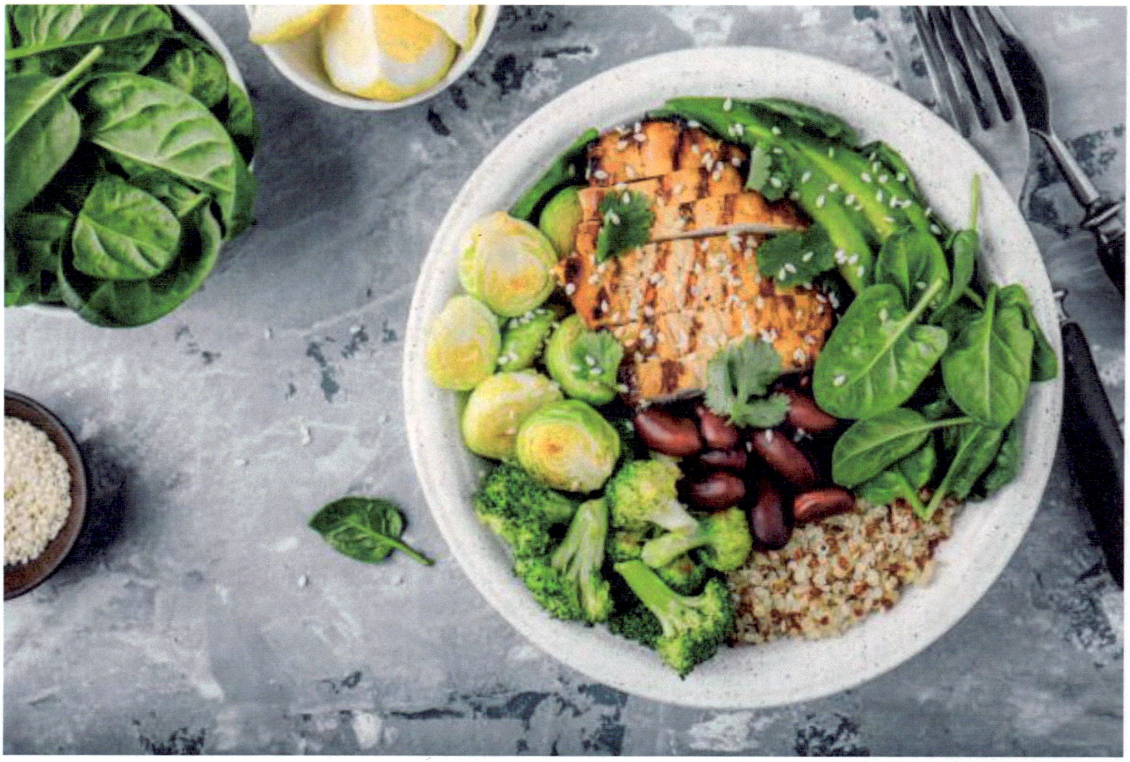

61. Chicken and Vegetable Quinoa Bowl

Prep.Time: 15 min

Cook Time: 25 min

Serving: 4

Beverage pairing: Green Tea

Ingredients:

- 1 cup quinoa, rinsed
- 2 cups chicken broth
- 2 boneless, skinless chicken breasts, cooked and shredded
- 2 cups mixed vegetables (such as bell peppers, broccoli, carrots)
- 2 tablespoons olive
- 2 cloves garlic, minced
- Salt and pepper to taste
- 2 tablespoons soy sauce or tamari
- 1 tablespoon honey or maple syrup
- 1 teaspoon sesame oil

Preparation:

1. In a saucepan, combine quinoa and chicken broth. Bring to a boil, then reduce heat to low, cover, and simmer for 15-20 minutes, or until quinoa is cooked and liquid is absorbed. Remove from heat and let it sit, covered, for 5 minutes. Fluff with a fork.
2. Heat olive oil in a large skillet or wok over medium-high heat.
3. Add minced garlic to the skillet. Cook until fragrant, about 1 minute.
4. Add mixed vegetables to the skillet. Stir-fry until tender-crisp, about 5-7 minutes.
5. Stir in cooked shredded chicken and cooked quinoa.
6. In a small bowl, whisk together soy sauce or tamari, honey or maple syrup, and sesame oil.
7. Pour the sauce over the chicken, vegetable, and quinoa mixture. Stir well to combine.
8. Cook for another 2-3 minutes until heated through.
9. Garnish with sesame seeds and chopped green onions if desired.
10. Serve chicken and vegetable quinoa bowls hot.

Nutrition Facts (per serving):

- Calories: 350
- Carbohydrates: 35g
- Protein: 30g
- Fat: 12g

62. Mediterranean Tofu Salad

Prep.Time: 15 min

Cook Time: 30 min

Serving: 4

Beverage pairing: Herbal Tea

Ingredients:

- 1 block extra-firm tofu, pressed and cubed
- 2 tablespoons olive oil
- 2 cloves garlic, minced
- 1 teaspoon dried oregano
- 1 teaspoon dried basil
- Salt and pepper to taste
- 4 cups mixed salad greens
- 1 cucumber, sliced
- 1 cup cherry tomatoes, halved
- 1/4 cup sliced Kalamata olives
- 1/4 cup crumbled feta cheese

Preparation:

1. Preheat oven to 400°F (200°C).
2. In a bowl, toss cubed tofu with olive oil, minced garlic, dried oregano, dried basil, salt, and pepper until evenly coated.
3. Spread tofu cubes in a single layer on a baking sheet lined with parchment paper.
4. Bake tofu in the preheated oven for 25-30 minutes, or until golden brown and crispy, flipping halfway through.
5. In a large salad bowl, combine mixed salad greens, sliced cucumber, halved cherry tomatoes, sliced Kalamata olives, and crumbled feta cheese.
6. In a small bowl, whisk together lemon juice, balsamic vinegar, and extra-virgin olive oil to make the dressing.
7. Drizzle the dressing over the salad and toss to coat evenly.
8. Top the salad with roasted tofu cubes.
9. Serve Mediterranean tofu salad immediately.

Nutrition Facts (per serving):

- Calories: 300
- Carbohydrates: 15g
- Protein: 15g
- Fat: 20g

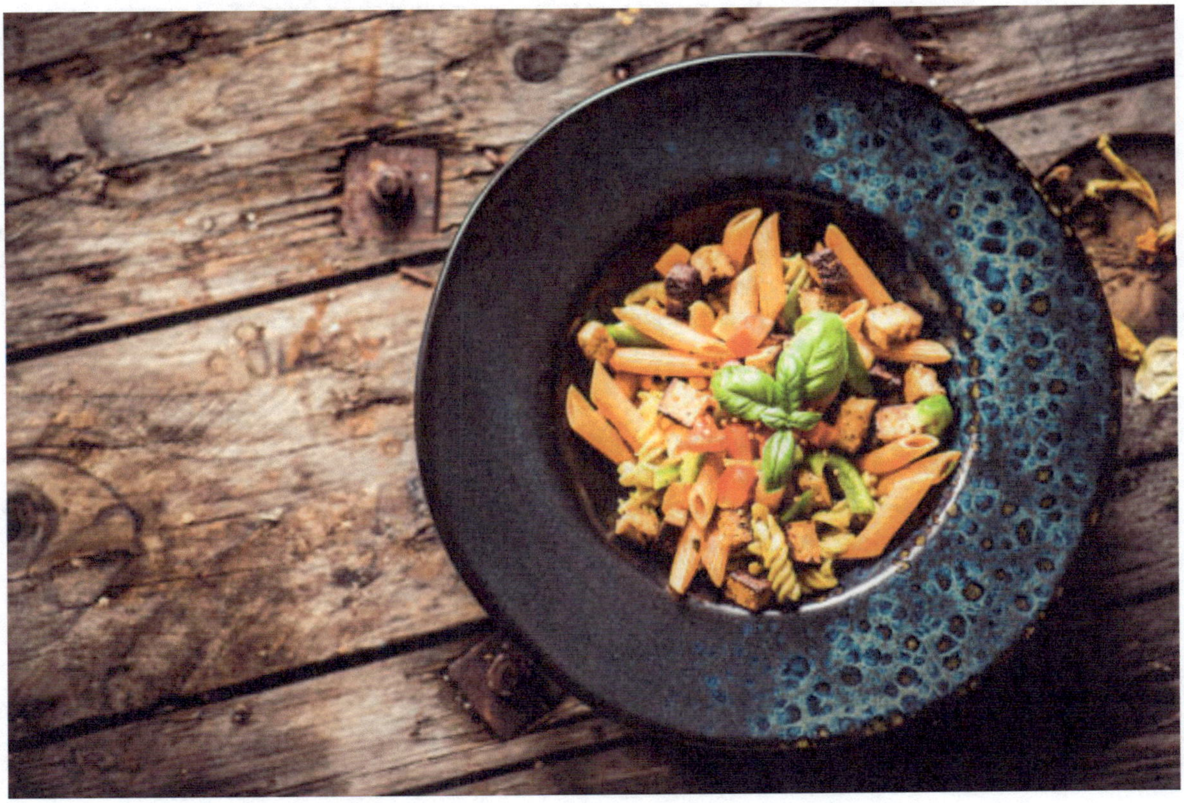

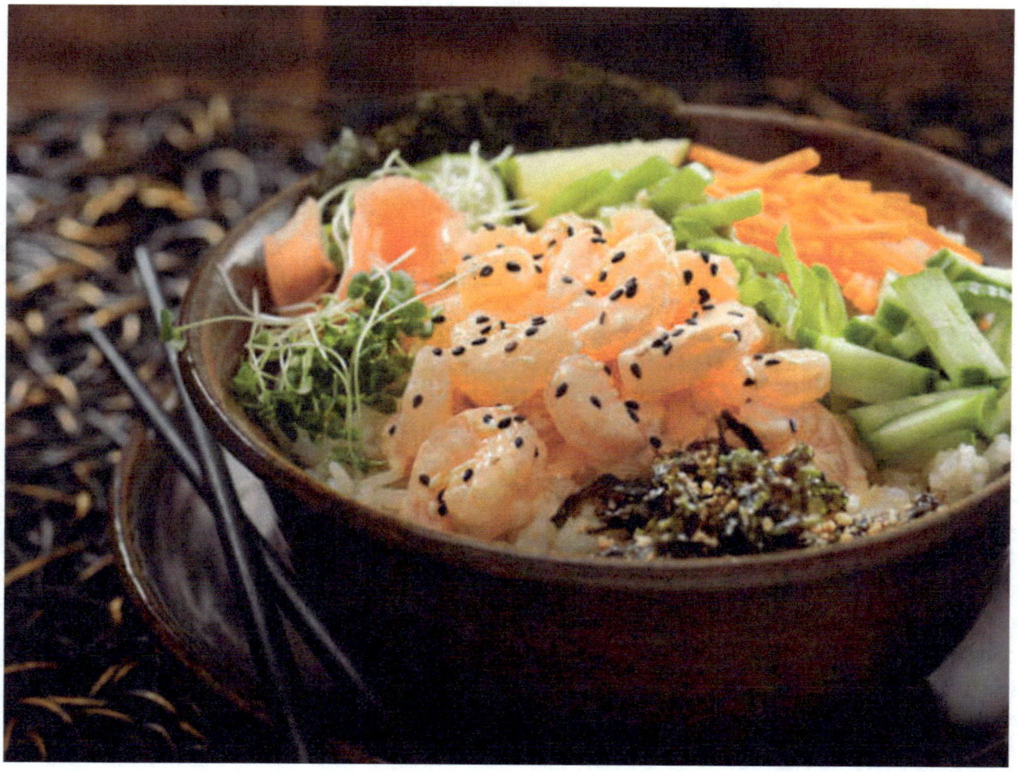

63. Shrimp and Avocado Quinoa Bowl

Prep.Time: 15 min

Cook Time: 20 min

Serving: 4

Beverage pairing: Iced Tea

Ingredients:

- 1 cup quinoa, rinsed
- 2 cups water or vegetable broth
- 1 lb shrimp, peeled and deveined
- 1 tablespoon olive oil
- 2 cloves garlic, minced
- 1 teaspoon smoked paprika
- Salt and pepper to taste
- 1 avocado, diced
- 1/4 cup diced red onion
- 1/4 cup chopped fresh cilantro
- Juice of 1 lime

Preparation:

1. In a saucepan, combine quinoa and water or vegetable broth. Bring to a boil, then reduce heat to low, cover, and simmer for 15-20 minutes, or until quinoa is cooked and liquid is absorbed. Remove from heat and let it sit, covered, for 5 minutes. Fluff with a fork.
2. Heat olive oil in a large skillet over medium heat.
3. Add minced garlic to the skillet. Cook until fragrant, about 1 minute.
4. Add shrimp to the skillet. Sprinkle with smoked paprika, salt, and pepper. Cook until shrimp turn pink and opaque, about 2-3 minutes per side.
5. In a large bowl, combine cooked quinoa, cooked shrimp, diced avocado, diced red onion, chopped fresh cilantro, and lime juice.
6. Toss gently to combine.
7. Serve shrimp and avocado quinoa bowls immediately.

Nutrition Facts (per serving):

- Calories: 350
- Carbohydrates: 30g
- Protein: 25g
- Fat: 15g

64. Turkey and Vegetable Skillet with Quinoa

Prep.Time: 15 min

Cook Time: 25 min

Serving: 4

Beverage pairing: Iced Tea

Ingredients:

- 1 cup quinoa, rinsed
- 2 cups chicken broth
- 1 lb ground turkey
- 1 tablespoon olive oil
- 1 onion, diced
- 2 cloves garlic, minced
- 2 cups mixed vegetables (such as bell peppers, zucchini, carrots)
- 1 teaspoon dried thyme
- 1 teaspoon dried oregano
- 1/4 cup chopped fresh parsley

Preparation:

1. In a saucepan, combine quinoa and chicken broth. Bring to a boil, then reduce heat to low, cover, and simmer for 15-20 minutes, or until quinoa is cooked and liquid is absorbed. Remove from heat and let it sit, covered, for 5 minutes. Fluff with a fork.
2. Heat olive oil in a large skillet over medium heat.
3. Add diced onion and minced garlic to the skillet. Cook until softened, about 2-3 minutes.
4. Add ground turkey to the skillet. Cook, breaking up the meat with a spatula, until browned and cooked through.
5. Stir in mixed vegetables, dried thyme, dried oregano, salt, and pepper. Cook until vegetables are tender, about 5-7 minutes.
6. Stir in cooked quinoa and chopped fresh parsley.
7. Cook for another 2-3 minutes until heated through.
8. Serve turkey and vegetable skillet with quinoa hot.

Nutrition Facts (per serving):

- Calories: 350
- Carbohydrates: 30g
- Protein: 25g
- Fat: 15g

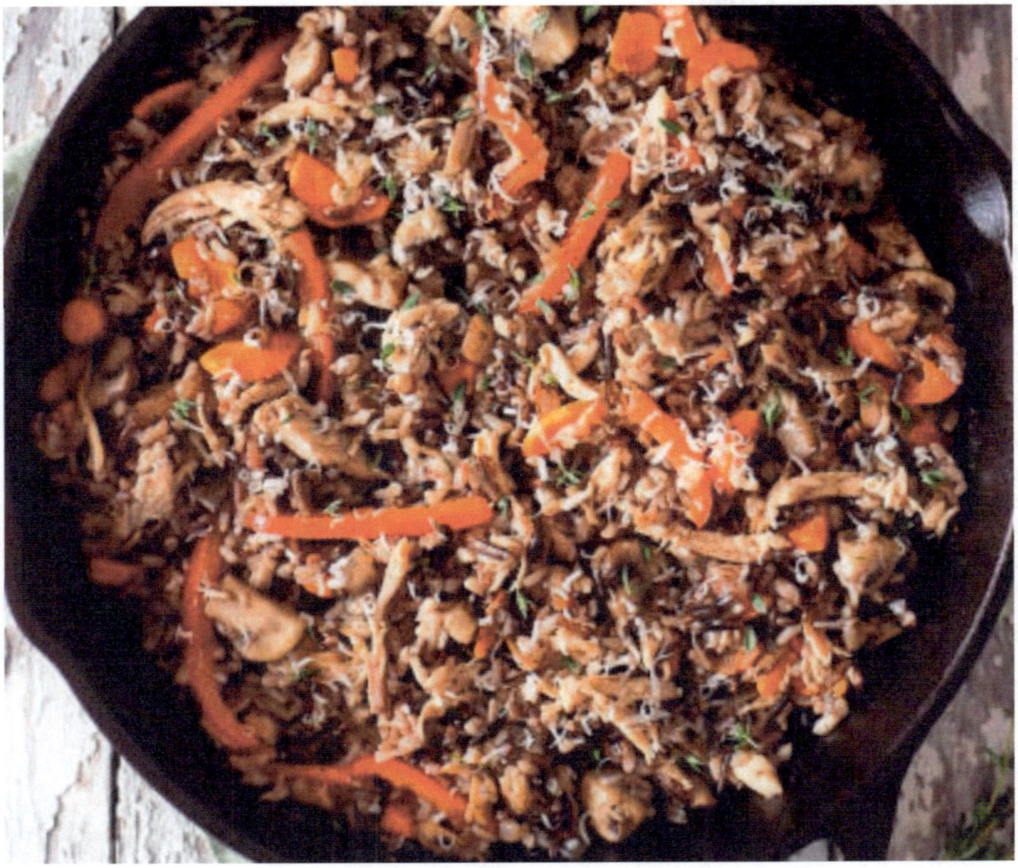

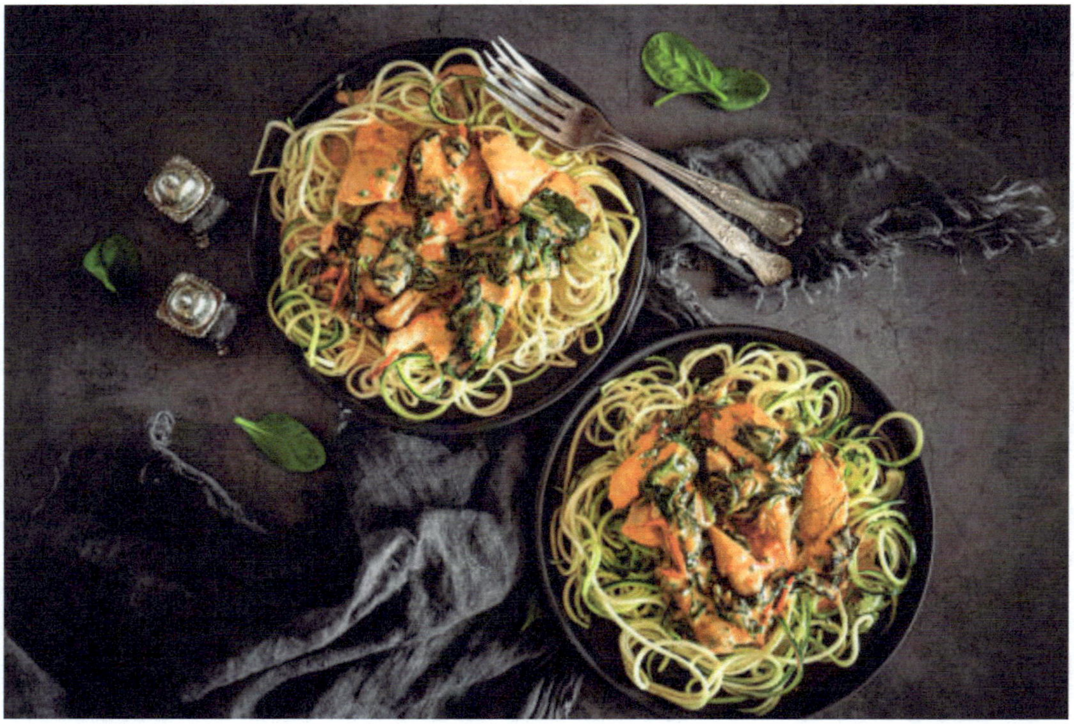

65. Caprese Chicken and Zucchini Noodle Bowl

Prep.Time:	Cook Time:	Serving:	Beverage pairing:
15 min	15 min	2	Lemonade

Ingredients:

- 2 boneless, skinless chicken breasts
- 2 tablespoons olive oil
- 2 cloves garlic, minced
- 2 large zucchinis, spiralized into noodles
- 1 cup cherry tomatoes, halved
- 1/2 cup fresh basil leaves, torn
- 4 oz fresh mozzarella cheese, sliced
- Balsamic glaze for drizzling
- Salt and pepper to taste

Preparation:

1. Season chicken breasts with salt and pepper.
2. Heat olive oil in a skillet over medium-high heat.
3. Add minced garlic to the skillet and cook until fragrant, about 1 minute.
4. Add chicken breasts to the skillet and cook for 6-7 minutes per side, or until cooked through and no longer pink in the center. Remove from heat and let rest for a few minutes before slicing.
5. In the same skillet, add spiralized zucchini noodles and cherry tomatoes. Cook for 2-3 minutes until slightly softened.
6. Divide zucchini noodles and cherry tomatoes into serving bowls.
7. Top with sliced chicken breasts, torn basil leaves, and fresh mozzarella slices.
8. Drizzle with balsamic glaze.
9. Serve Caprese chicken and zucchini noodle bowls immediately.

Nutrition Facts (per serving):

- Calories: 350
- Carbohydrates: 10g
- Protein: 30g
- Fat: 20g

66. Lentil and Mushroom Burgers

Prep.Time: 15 min

Cook Time: 10 min

Serving: 4

Beverage pairing: Herbal Tea

Ingredients:

- 1 cup cooked lentils
- 1 cup chopped mushrooms
- 1/2 cup rolled oats
- 1/4 cup chopped onion
- 2 cloves garlic, minced
- 1 teaspoon ground cumin
- 1 teaspoon smoked paprika
- Salt and pepper to taste
- Olive oil for cooking

Preparation:

1. In a food processor, pulse cooked lentils, chopped mushrooms, rolled oats, chopped onion, minced garlic, ground cumin, smoked paprika, salt, and pepper until well combined but still slightly chunky.
2. Form the mixture into burger patties.
3. Heat olive oil in a skillet over medium heat.
4. Cook lentil and mushroom burgers for 4-5 minutes per side, or until golden brown and heated through.
5. Serve lentil and mushroom burgers on whole wheat burger buns with your favorite toppings.

Nutrition Facts (per serving, without bun and toppings):

- Calories: 200
- Carbohydrates: 30g
- Protein: 10g
- Fat: 5g

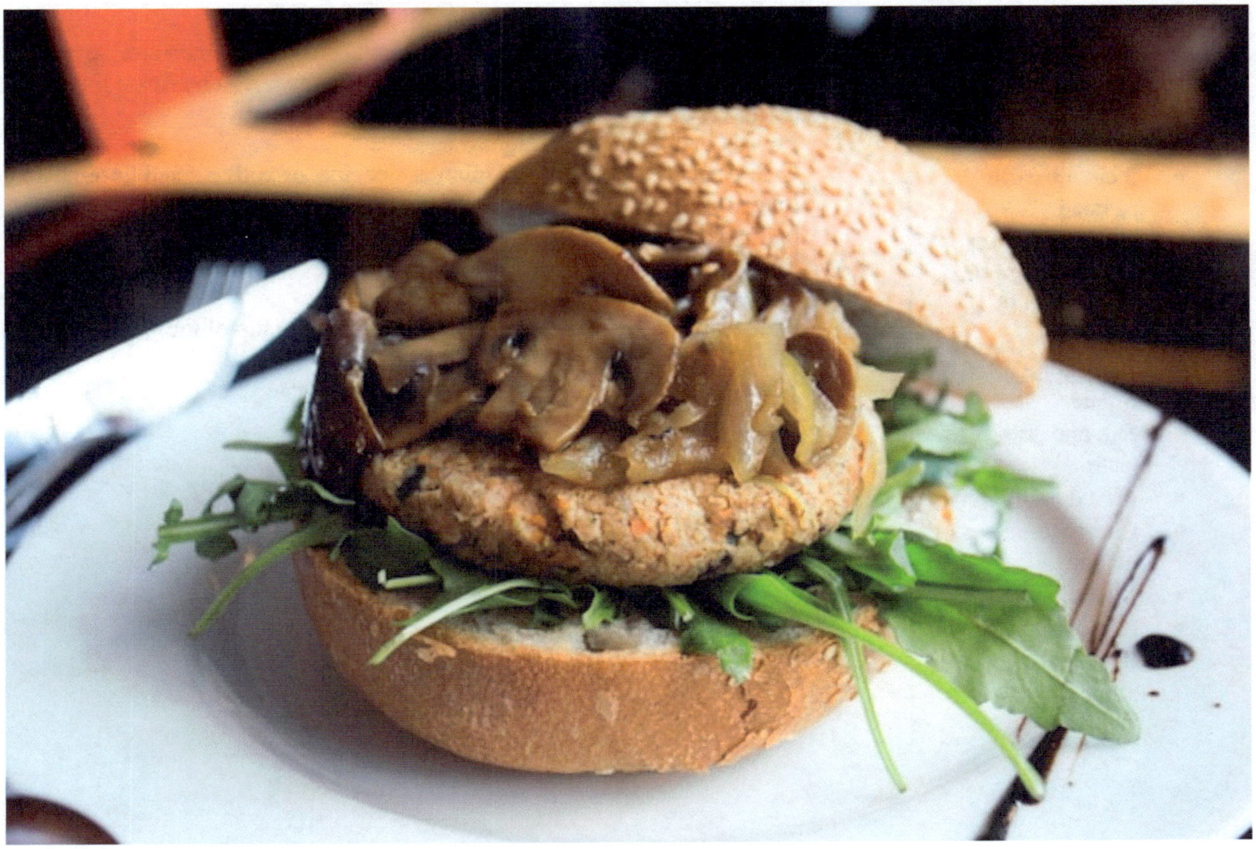

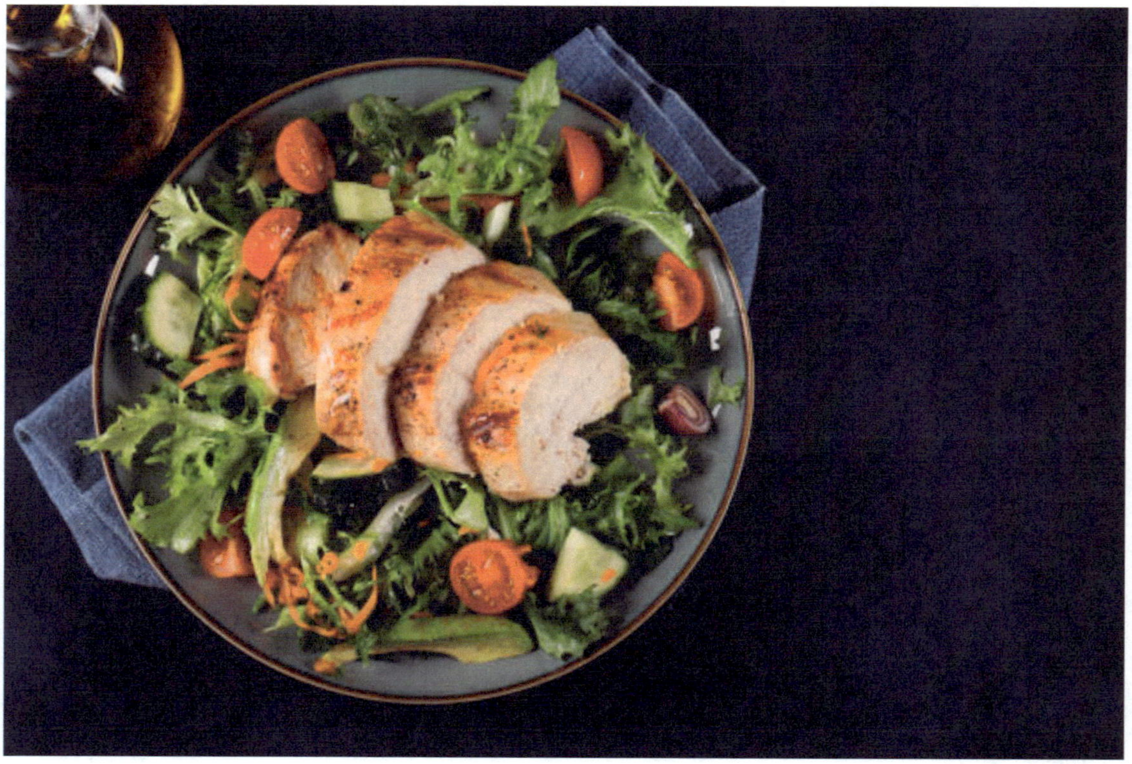

67. Grilled Lemon Herb Chicken Salad

Prep.Time: 10 min

Cook Time: 15 min

Serving: 2

Beverage pairing: Mint Water

Ingredients:

- 2 boneless, skinless chicken breasts
- 2 tablespoons olive oil
- 2 cloves garlic, minced
- Zest of 1 lemon
- Juice of 1 lemon
- 1 teaspoon dried oregano
- 1 teaspoon dried thyme
- Salt and pepper to taste
- Mixed salad greens
- Cherry tomatoes, halved
- Cucumber slices
- Red onion slices
- Balsamic vinaigrette for dressing

Preparation:

1. Season chicken breasts with olive oil, minced garlic, lemon zest, lemon juice, dried oregano, dried thyme, salt, and pepper. Let marinate for at least 30 minutes.
2. Preheat grill to medium-high heat.
3. Grill chicken breasts for 6-7 minutes per side, or until cooked through and no longer pink in the center. Remove from heat and let rest for a few minutes before slicing.
4. In a large salad bowl, combine mixed salad greens, cherry tomatoes, cucumber slices, and red onion slices.
5. Slice grilled chicken breasts and arrange them on top of the salad.
6. Drizzle with balsamic vinaigrette.
7. Serve grilled lemon herb chicken salad immediately.

Nutrition Facts (per serving):

- Calories: 300
- Carbohydrates: 10g
- Protein: 30g
- Fat: 15g

68. Asian-inspired Salmon and Broccoli Bowl

Prep.Time: 10 min

Cook Time: 15 min

Serving: 2

Beverage pairing: Green Tea

Ingredients:

- 2 salmon fillets
- 2 tablespoons soy sauce or tamari
- 1 tablespoon honey or maple syrup
- 1 clove garlic, minced
- 1 teaspoon grated ginger
- 2 cups broccoli florets
- 1 tablespoon olive oil
- Cooked brown rice for serving
- Sesame seeds for garnish (optional)
- Sliced green onions for garnish (optional)

Preparation:

1. Preheat oven to 400°F (200°C).
2. In a small bowl, whisk together soy sauce or tamari, honey or maple syrup, minced garlic, and grated ginger to make the marinade.
3. Place salmon fillets in a shallow dish and pour the marinade over them. Let marinate for at least 15 minutes.
4. Place broccoli florets on a baking sheet lined with parchment paper. Drizzle with olive oil and season with salt and pepper.
5. Arrange marinated salmon fillets on the baking sheet with broccoli florets.
6. Bake in the preheated oven for 12-15 minutes, or until salmon is cooked through and flakes easily with a fork.
7. Divide cooked brown rice into serving bowls.
8. Top with baked salmon fillets and roasted broccoli florets.
9. Garnish with sesame seeds and sliced green onions if desired.
10. Serve Asian-inspired salmon and broccoli bowls hot.

Nutrition Facts (per serving):

- Calories: 400
- Carbohydrates: 30g
- Protein: 30g
- Fat: 18g

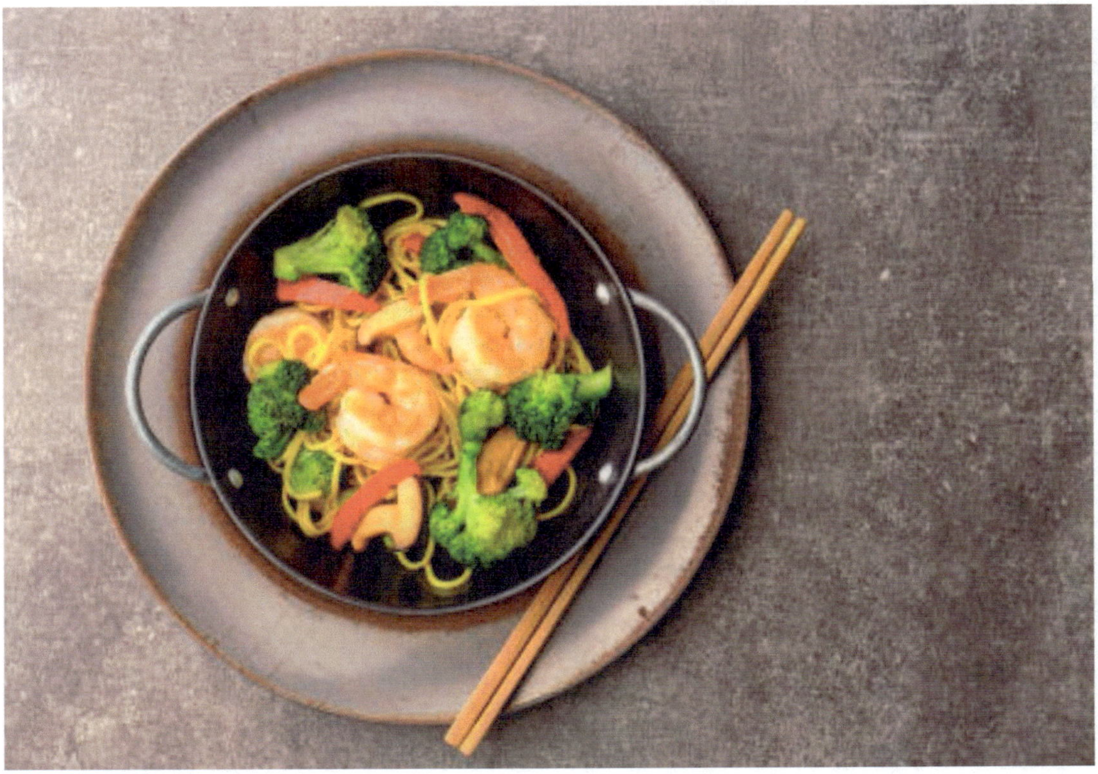

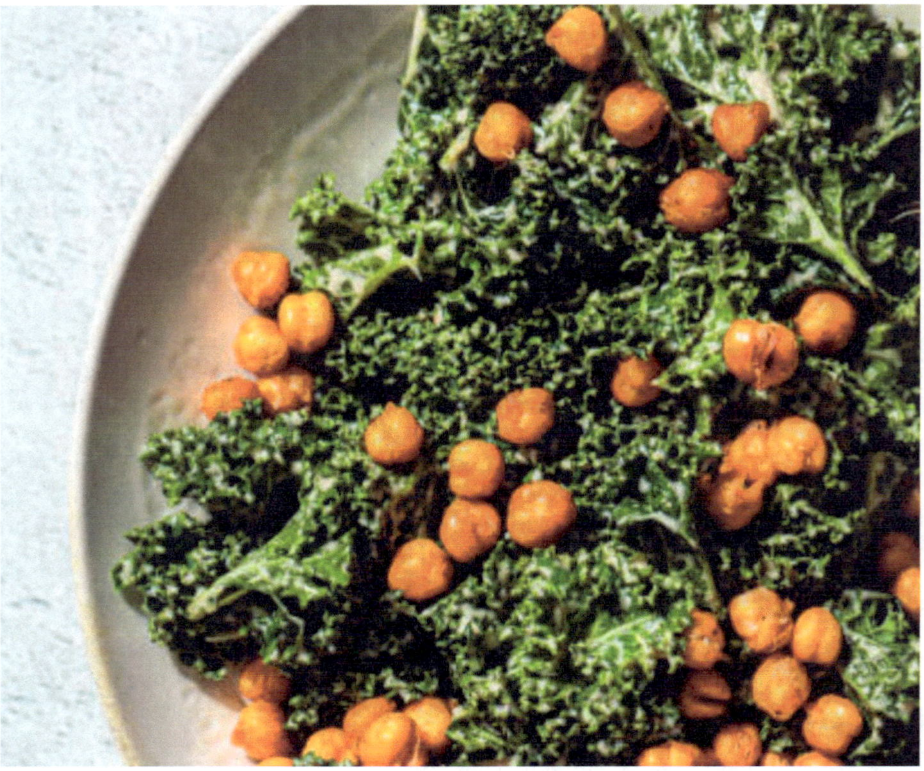

69. Chickpea and Kale Caesar Salad

Prep.Time: 10 min

Cook Time: 25 min

Serving: 4

Beverage pairing: Mint Water

Ingredients:

- 1 can (15 oz) chickpeas, drained and rinsed
- 4 cups chopped kale leaves
- 2 tablespoons olive oil
- 1 tablespoon lemon juice
- 1 clove garlic, minced
- 1/4 cup grated Parmesan cheese
- Salt and pepper to taste
- Caesar dressing (store-bought or homemade)
- Croutons for garnish (optional)

Preparation:

1. Preheat oven to 400°F (200°C).
2. Spread chickpeas in a single layer on a baking sheet lined with parchment paper.
3. Drizzle chickpeas with olive oil and lemon juice. Sprinkle minced garlic, grated Parmesan cheese, salt, and pepper over the chickpeas.
4. Roast chickpeas in the preheated oven for 20-25 minutes, or until golden and crispy.
5. In a large salad bowl, massage chopped kale leaves with a drizzle of olive oil for a few minutes until softened.
6. Add roasted chickpeas to the salad bowl.
7. Drizzle Caesar dressing over the salad and toss to coat evenly.
8. Garnish with croutons if desired.
9. Serve chickpea and kale Caesar salad immediately.

Nutrition Facts (per serving):

- Calories: 300
- Carbohydrates: 20g
- Protein: 12g
- Fat: 18g

70. Turkey and Spinach Stuffed Mushrooms

Prep.Time: 15 min

Cook Time: 12 min

Serving: 4

Beverage pairing: Lemonade

Ingredients:

- 12 large mushrooms, stems removed and reserved
- 1/2 lb ground turkey
- 1/4 cup diced onion
- 1 clove garlic, minced
- 1 cup chopped spinach
- 1/4 cup grated Parmesan cheese
- Salt and pepper to taste
- Olive oil for brushing

Preparation:

1. Preheat oven to 375°F (190°C).
2. Finely chop the reserved mushroom stems.
3. Heat olive oil in a skillet over medium heat.
4. Add diced onion and minced garlic to the skillet. Cook until softened, about 2-3 minutes.
5. Add ground turkey to the skillet. Cook until browned and cooked through, breaking up the meat with a spatula.
6. Stir in chopped mushroom stems and chopped spinach. Cook for another 2-3 minutes until spinach wilts.
7. Remove skillet from heat and stir in grated Parmesan cheese. Season with salt and pepper to taste. Brush the outside of each mushroom cap with olive oil. Stuff each mushroom cap with the turkey and spinach mixture.
8. Place stuffed mushrooms on a baking sheet lined with parchment paper.
9. Bake in the preheated oven for 15-20 minutes, or until mushrooms are tender and filling is heated through.
10. Serve turkey and spinach stuffed mushrooms hot.

Nutrition Facts (per serving, 3 mushrooms):

- Calories: 200
- Carbohydrates: 5g
- Protein: 20g
- Fat: 10g

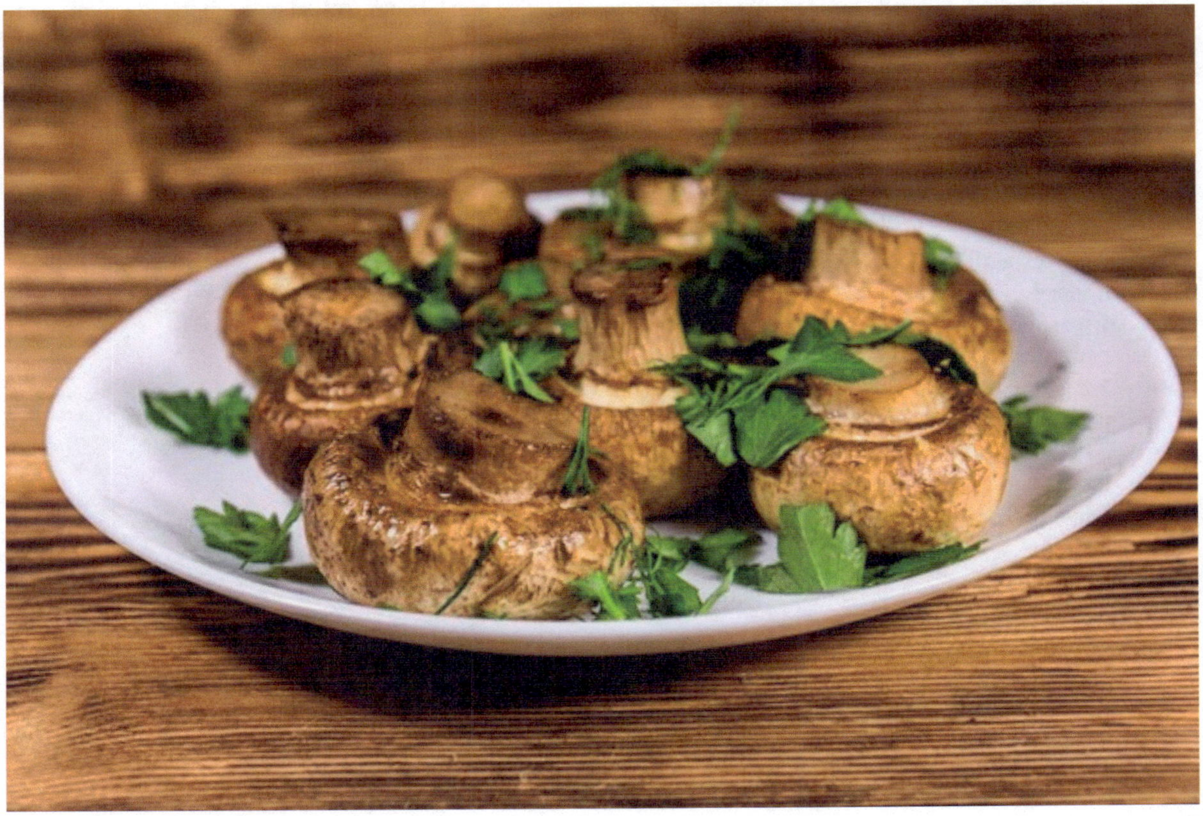

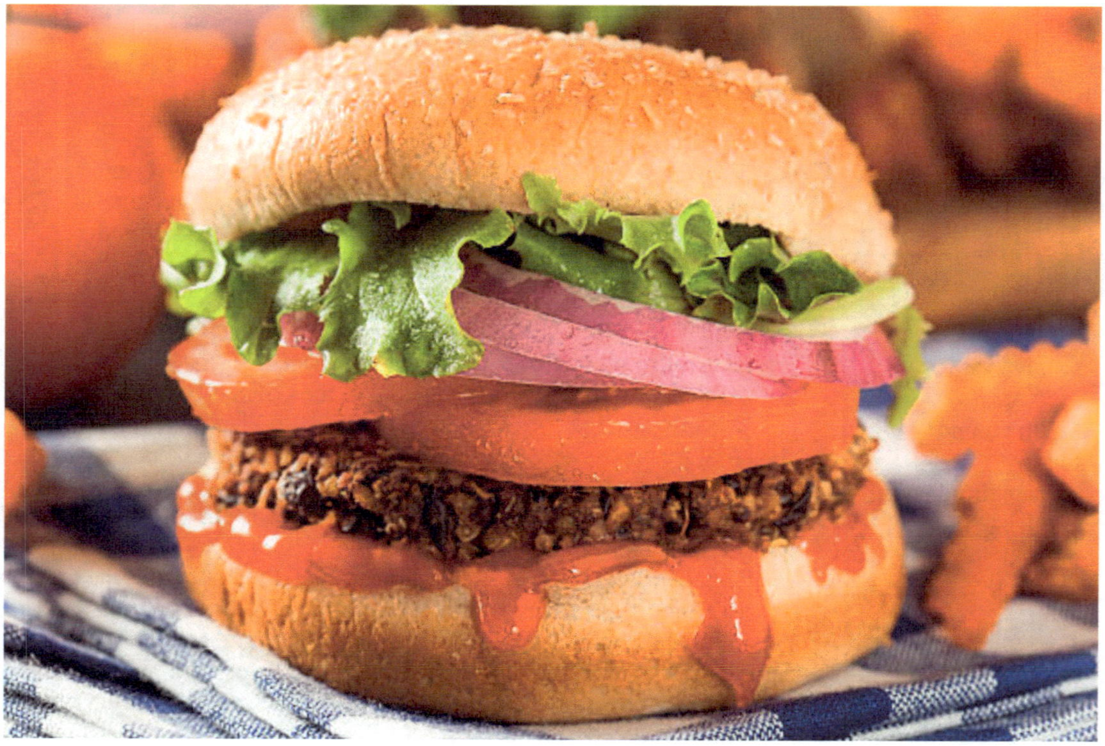

71. Quinoa and Black Bean Veggie Burger

Prep.Time: 15 min

Cook Time: 10 min

Serving: 4

Beverage pairing: Herbal Tea

Ingredients:

- 1 cup cooked quinoa
- 1 can (15 oz) black beans, drained and rinsed
- 1/2 cup rolled oats
- 1/4 cup chopped onion
- 2 cloves garlic, minced
- 1 teaspoon ground cumin
- 1 teaspoon chili powder
- Salt and pepper to taste
- Olive oil for cooking

Preparation:

1. In a food processor, pulse black beans, rolled oats, chopped onion, minced garlic, ground cumin, chili powder, salt, and pepper until well combined but still slightly chunky.
2. Transfer the mixture to a bowl and stir in cooked quinoa until evenly distributed.
3. Form the mixture into burger patties.
4. Heat olive oil in a skillet over medium heat.
5. Cook quinoa and black bean veggie burgers for 4-5 minutes per side, or until golden brown and heated through.
6. Serve veggie burgers on whole wheat burger buns with your favorite toppings.

Nutrition Facts (per serving, without bun and toppings):

- Calories: 200
- Carbohydrates: 30g
- Protein: 10g
- Fat: 5g

72. Chicken and Vegetable Stir-Fry with Cauliflower Rice

Prep.Time: 15 min

Cook Time: 15 min

Serving: 4

Beverage pairing: Lemonade

Ingredients:

- 2 boneless, skinless chicken breasts, thinly sliced
- 2 tablespoons soy sauce or tamari
- 1 tablespoon oyster sauce (optional)
- 1 tablespoon sesame oil
- 2 tablespoons olive oil
- 2 cloves garlic, minced
- 1 teaspoon grated ginger
- 2 cups mixed vegetables (such as bell peppers, broccoli, carrots)
- 1 head cauliflower, riced

Preparation:

1. In a bowl, combine sliced chicken breasts, soy sauce or tamari, and oyster sauce (if using). Let marinate for at least 15 minutes.
2. Heat sesame oil and olive oil in a large skillet or wok over medium-high heat.
3. Add minced garlic and grated ginger to the skillet. Cook until fragrant, about 1 minute.
4. Add marinated chicken slices to the skillet. Stir-fry until chicken is cooked through, about 5-7 minutes.
5. Stir in mixed vegetables and continue to stir-fry for another 3-4 minutes until vegetables are tender-crisp.
6. Push chicken and vegetables to one side of the skillet. Add riced cauliflower to the empty side of the skillet.
7. Cook cauliflower rice for 2-3 minutes, stirring occasionally, until heated through.
8. Season chicken, vegetables, and cauliflower rice with salt and pepper to taste. Garnish with chopped green onions and sesame seeds if desired.
9. Serve chicken and vegetable stir-fry with cauliflower rice hot.

Nutrition Facts (per serving):

- Calories: 300
- Carbohydrates: 15g
- Protein: 25g
- Fat: 15g

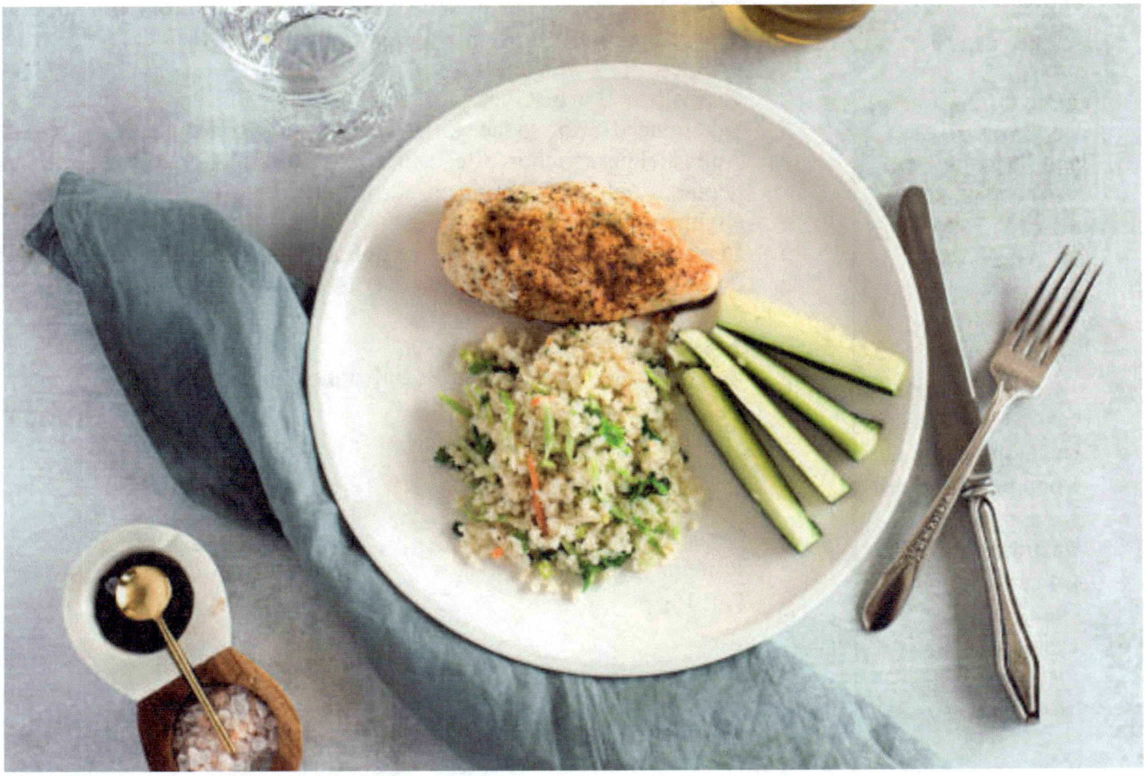

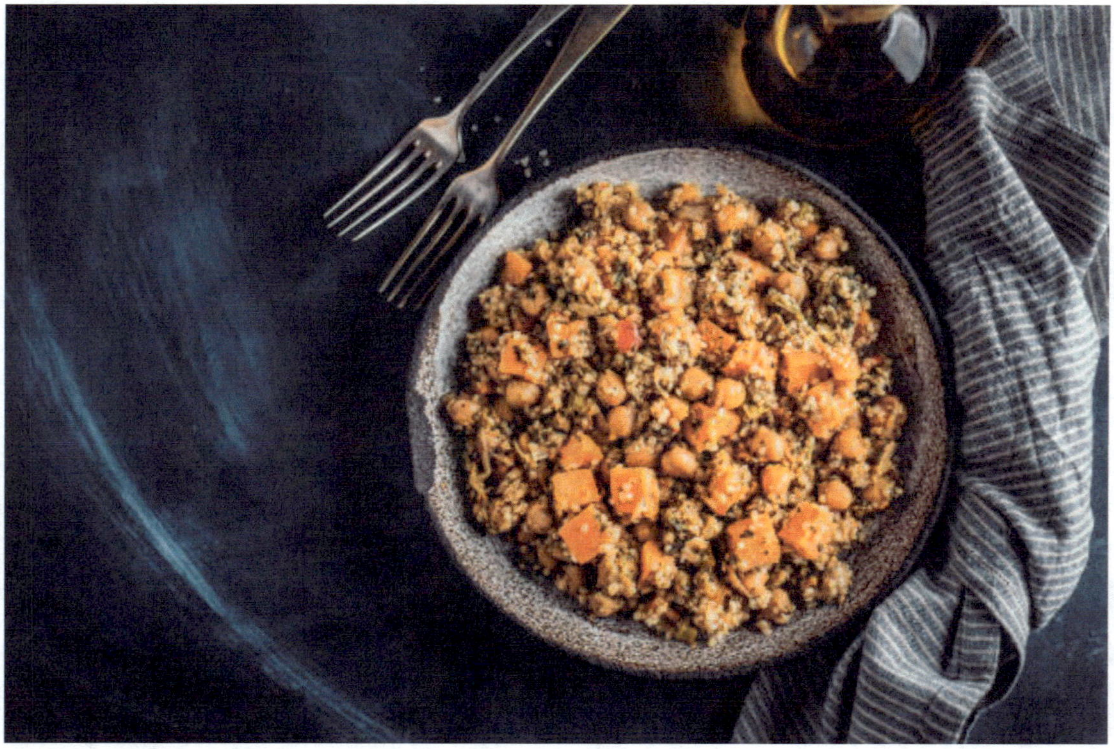

73. Mediterranean Chickpea and Quinoa Bowl

Prep.Time: 15 min

Cook Time: 20 min

Serving: 4

Beverage pairing: Mint Water

Ingredients:

- 1 cup quinoa, rinsed
- 2 cups vegetable broth
- 1 can (15 oz) chickpeas, drained and rinsed
- 2 tablespoons olive oil
- 2 cloves garlic, minced
- 1 teaspoon dried oregano
- 1 teaspoon dried basil
- 1 cucumber, diced
- 1 bell pepper, diced
- 1/4 cup sliced Kalamata olives
- 1/4 cup crumbled feta cheese
- 2 tablespoons chopped fresh parsley

Preparation:

1. In a saucepan, combine quinoa and vegetable broth. Bring to a boil, then reduce heat to low, cover, and simmer for 15-20 minutes, or until quinoa is cooked and liquid is absorbed. Remove from heat and let it sit, covered, for 5 minutes. Fluff with a fork.
2. Heat olive oil in a skillet over medium heat.
3. Add minced garlic to the skillet. Cook until fragrant, about 1 minute.
4. Add chickpeas to the skillet. Stir in dried oregano, dried basil, salt, and pepper. Cook for 5-7 minutes, stirring occasionally, until chickpeas are slightly crispy.
5. In a large bowl, combine cooked quinoa, sautéed chickpeas, diced cucumber, diced bell pepper, sliced Kalamata olives, crumbled feta cheese, lemon juice, and chopped fresh parsley.
6. Toss gently to combine.
7. Serve Mediterranean chickpea and quinoa bowls immediately.

Nutrition Facts (per serving):

- Calories: 350
- Carbohydrates: 45g
- Protein: 12g
- Fat: 15g

74. Turkey and Avocado Caesar Wrap

Prep.Time: 10 min | **Cook Time:** 0 min | **Serving:** 4 | **Beverage pairing:** Iced Tea

Ingredients:

- 4 whole wheat wraps or tortillas
- 1 lb cooked turkey breast, sliced
- 1 avocado, sliced
- 2 cups shredded romaine lettuce
- 1/4 cup grated Parmesan cheese
- Caesar dressing (store-bought or homemade)
- Salt and pepper to taste

Preparation:

1. Lay out the whole wheat wraps or tortillas on a flat surface.
2. Divide the sliced turkey breast, avocado slices, shredded romaine lettuce, and grated Parmesan cheese evenly among the wraps.
3. Drizzle Caesar dressing over the ingredients on each wrap.
4. Season with salt and pepper to taste.
5. Tightly roll up each wrap, folding in the sides as you go.
6. Cut the wraps in half diagonally before serving, if desired.
7. Serve turkey and avocado Caesar wraps immediately.

Nutrition Facts (per serving):

- Calories: 350
- Carbohydrates: 30g
- Protein: 25g
- Fat: 15g

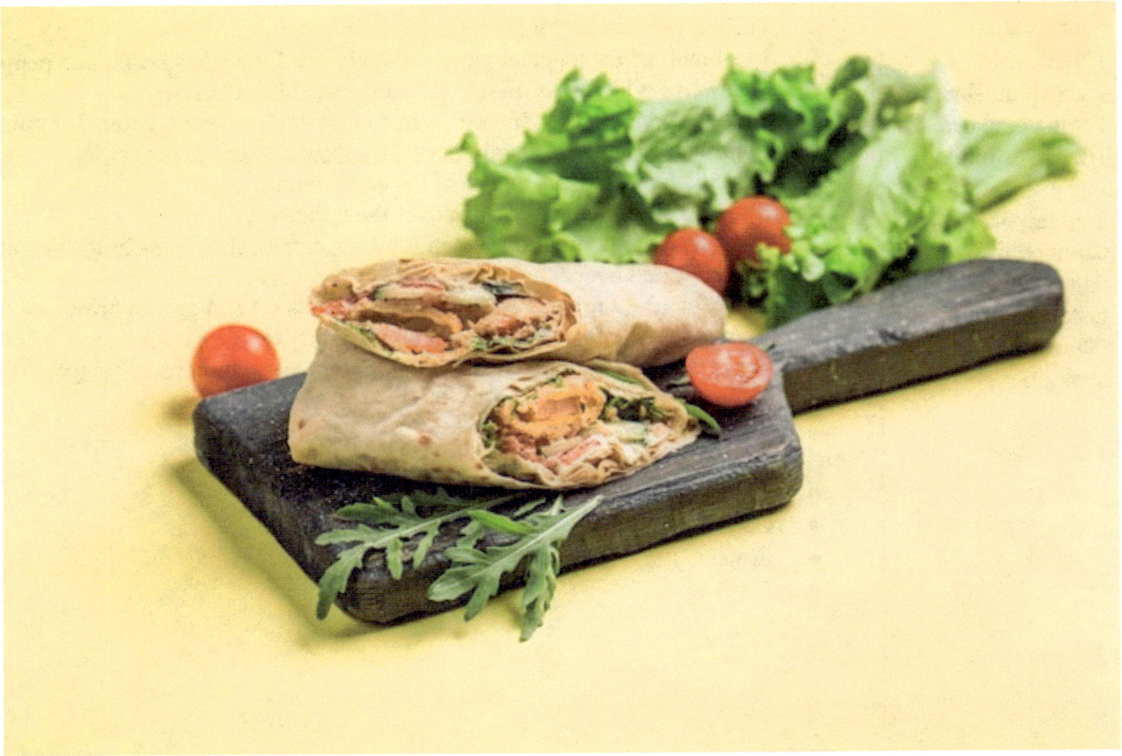

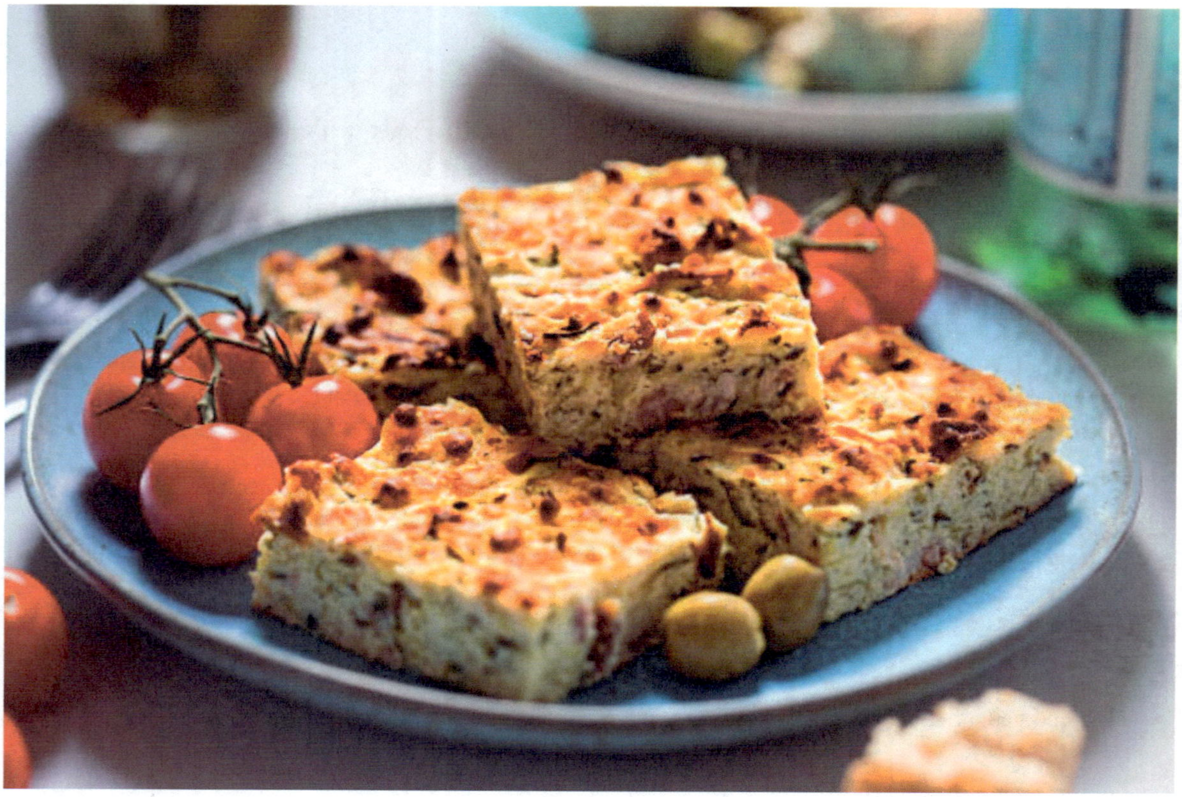

75. Zucchini and Tomato Frittata with Feta

Prep.Time: 10 min

Cook Time: 20 min

Serving: 4

Beverage pairing: Lemonade

Ingredients:

- 6 large eggs
- 1/4 cup milk
- 1 zucchini, sliced
- 1 tomato, sliced
- 1/2 cup crumbled feta cheese
- 2 tablespoons chopped fresh basil
- Salt and pepper to taste
- Olive oil for cooking

Preparation:

1. Preheat oven to 350°F (175°C).
2. In a bowl, whisk together eggs, milk, chopped fresh basil, salt, and pepper.
3. Heat olive oil in an oven-safe skillet over medium heat.
4. Add zucchini slices to the skillet and cook until softened, about 3-4 minutes.
5. Pour the egg mixture evenly over the zucchini slices in the skillet.
6. Arrange tomato slices on top of the egg mixture.
7. Sprinkle crumbled feta cheese over the tomatoes.
8. Cook the frittata on the stovetop for 2-3 minutes, then transfer the skillet to the preheated oven.
9. Bake for 10-12 minutes, or until the frittata is set and golden brown on top.
10. Remove from the oven and let it cool slightly before slicing.
11. Serve zucchini and tomato frittata with feta warm or at room temperature.

Nutrition Facts (per serving):

- Calories: 200
- Carbohydrates: 5g
- Protein: 12g
- Fat: 15g

76. Lentil and Vegetable Stuffed Pita

Prep.Time: 10 min

Cook Time: 0 min

Serving: 4

Beverage pairing: Herbal Tea

Ingredients:

- 4 whole wheat pitas, halved
- 1 cup cooked lentils
- 1 cup diced cucumber
- 1 cup diced tomatoes
- 1/2 cup diced red onion
- 1/4 cup chopped fresh parsley
- Juice of 1 lemon
- 2 tablespoons extra-virgin olive oil
- Salt and pepper to taste
- Hummus for spreading (optional)

Preparation:

1. In a large bowl, combine cooked lentils, diced cucumber, diced tomatoes, diced red onion, chopped fresh parsley, lemon juice, extra-virgin olive oil, salt, and pepper. Toss to combine.
2. Warm the whole wheat pitas in the microwave or oven until slightly soft.
3. Spread a spoonful of hummus (if using) on the inside of each pita half.
4. Fill each pita half with the lentil and vegetable mixture.
5. Serve lentil and vegetable stuffed pitas immediately.

Nutrition Facts (per serving):

- Calories: 250
- Carbohydrates: 40g
- Protein: 10g
- Fat: 5g

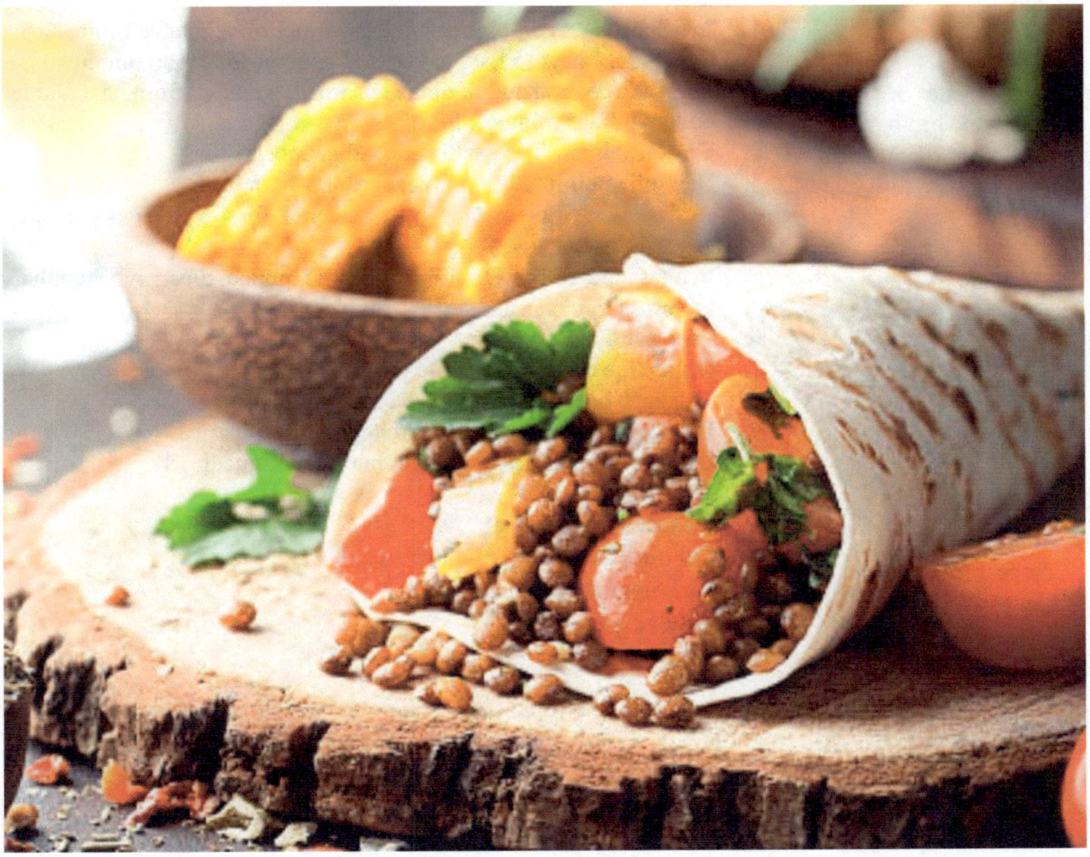

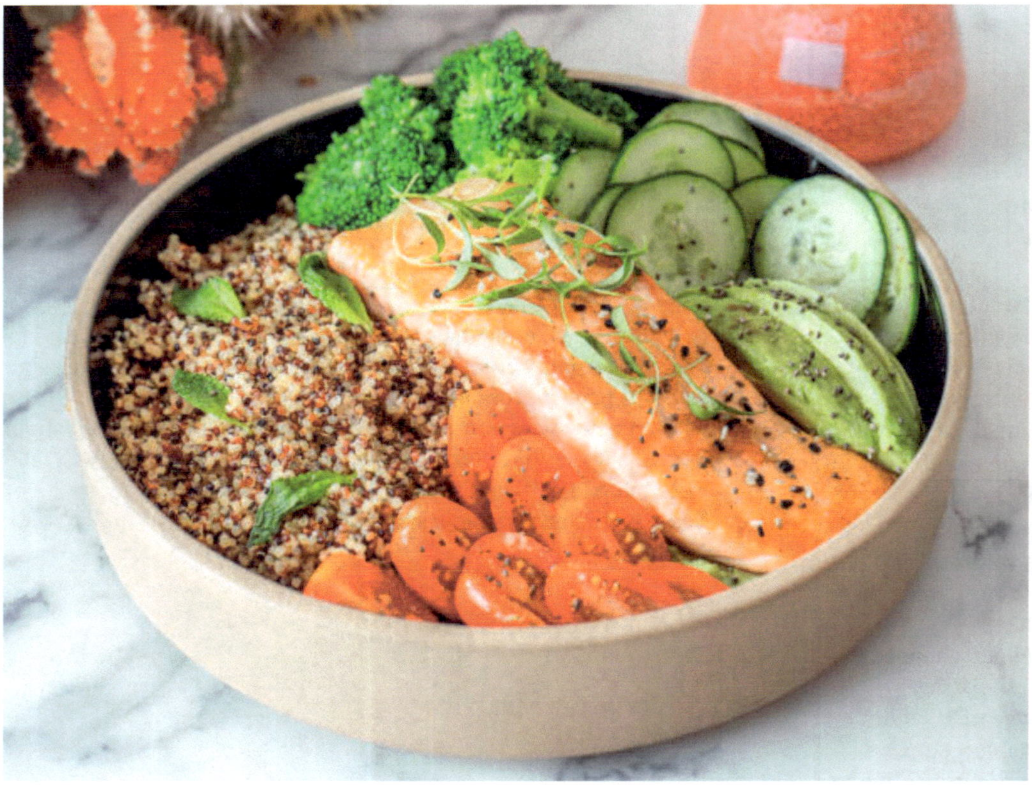

77. Salmon and Avocado Quinoa Salad

Prep.Time: 15 min | **Cook Time:** 20 min | **Serving:** 2 | **Beverage pairing:** Lemonade

Ingredients:

- 1 cup quinoa, rinsed
- 2 cups water or vegetable broth
- 2 salmon fillets
- 1 tablespoon olive oil
- 1 avocado, diced
- 1 cup cherry tomatoes, halved
- 2 cups mixed salad greens
- Juice of 1 lemon
- Salt and pepper to taste
- Balsamic vinaigrette for dressing

Preparation:

1. In a saucepan, combine quinoa and water or vegetable broth. Bring to a boil, then reduce heat to low, cover, and simmer for 15-20 minutes, or until quinoa is cooked and liquid is absorbed. Remove from heat and let it sit, covered, for 5 minutes. Fluff with a fork.
2. Season salmon fillets with salt and pepper.
3. Heat olive oil in a skillet over medium-high heat.
4. Add salmon fillets to the skillet and cook for 4-5 minutes per side, or until cooked through and flaky.
5. In a large salad bowl, combine cooked quinoa, diced avocado, halved cherry tomatoes, mixed salad greens, and lemon juice.
6. Toss gently to combine.
7. Divide the quinoa salad into serving bowls.
8. Top each bowl with a cooked salmon fillet.
9. Drizzle with balsamic vinaigrette.
10. Serve salmon and avocado quinoa salad immediately.

Nutrition Facts (per serving):

- Calories: 400
- Carbohydrates: 30g
- Protein: 30g
- Fat: 20g

78. Spinach and Feta Turkey Meatballs with Greek Yogurt Sauce

Prep.Time: 15 min

Cook Time: 25 min

Serving: 4

Beverage pairing: Herbal Tea

Ingredients:

- 1 lb ground turkey
- 1/2 cup chopped spinach
- 1/4 cup crumbled feta cheese
- 1/4 cup breadcrumbs
- 1 egg
- 2 cloves garlic, minced
- 1 teaspoon dried oregano
- Olive oil for cooking
- 1 cup Greek yogurt
- 1 tablespoon lemon juice
- 1 tablespoon chopped fresh dill

Preparation:

1. Preheat oven to 400°F (200°C). Line a baking sheet with parchment paper.
2. In a large bowl, combine ground turkey, chopped spinach, crumbled feta cheese, breadcrumbs, egg, minced garlic, dried oregano, salt, and pepper. Mix until well combined.
3. Roll the mixture into golf ball-sized meatballs and place them on the prepared baking sheet.
4. Bake in the preheated oven for 20-25 minutes, or until meatballs are cooked through and browned on the outside.
5. In the meantime, prepare the Greek yogurt sauce by mixing together Greek yogurt, lemon juice, chopped fresh dill, salt, and pepper in a small bowl.
6. Serve spinach and feta turkey meatballs hot with Greek yogurt sauce for dipping.

Nutrition Facts (per serving, 3 meatballs with sauce):

- Calories: 300
- Carbohydrates: 5g
- Protein: 30g
- Fat: 15g

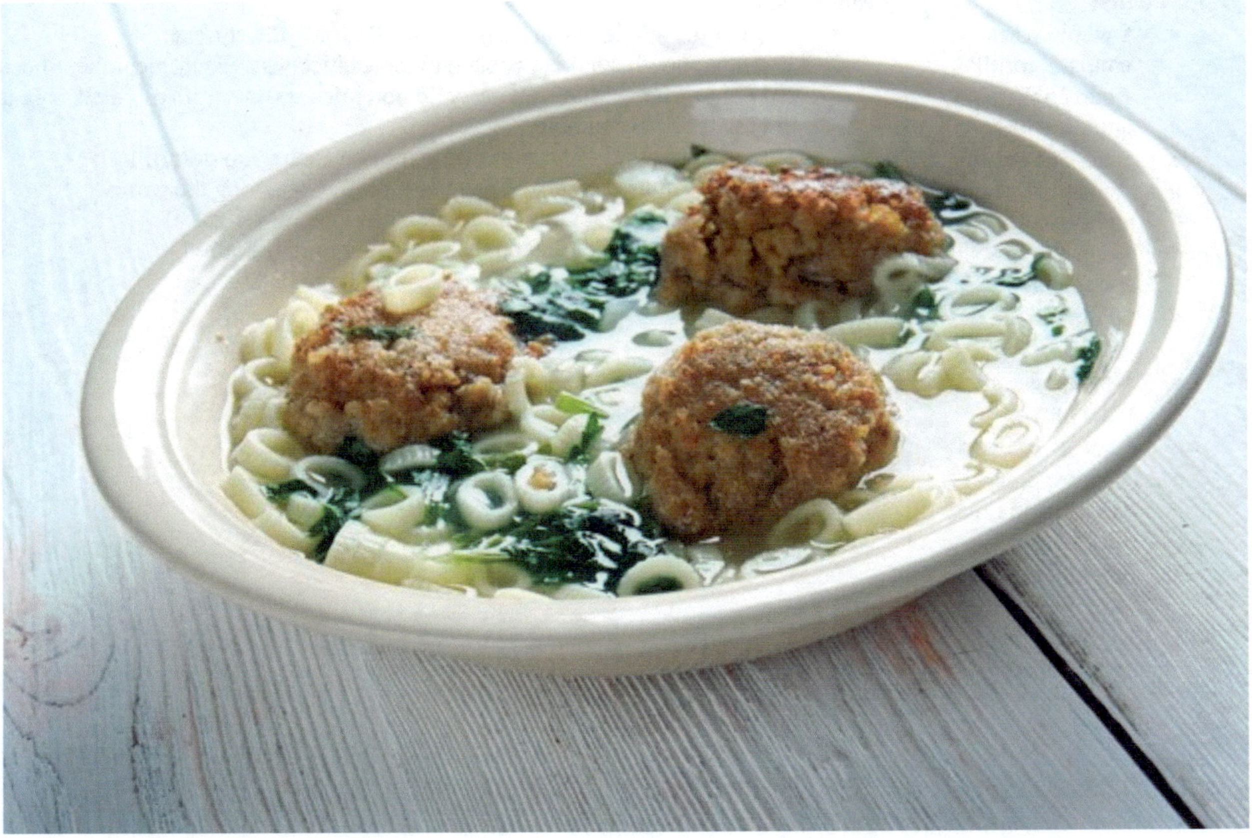

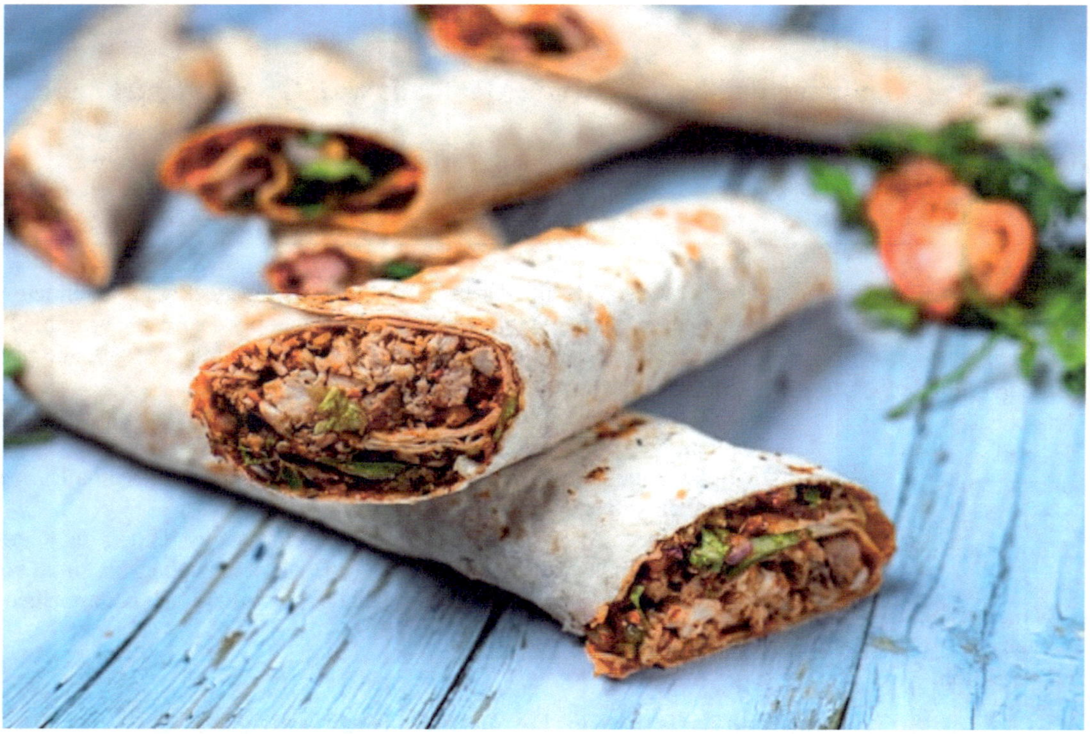

79. Greek Chickpea and Quinoa Wrap

Prep.Time: 10 min

Cook Time: 0 min

Serving: 4

Beverage pairing: Mint Water

Ingredients:

- 4 whole wheat wraps or tortillas
- 1 cup cooked quinoa
- 1 can (15 oz) chickpeas, drained and rinsed
- 1 cup diced cucumber
- 1/2 cup diced red onion
- 1/4 cup chopped fresh parsley
- Juice of 1 lemon
- 2 tablespoons extra-virgin olive oil
- Salt and pepper to taste
- Hummus for spreading (optional)

Preparation:

1. Lay out the whole wheat wraps or tortillas on a flat surface.
2. In a large bowl, combine cooked quinoa, chickpeas, diced cucumber, diced red onion, chopped fresh parsley, lemon juice, extra-virgin olive oil, salt, and pepper. Toss to combine.
3. Spread a spoonful of hummus (if using) on each wrap or tortilla.
4. Divide the quinoa and chickpea mixture evenly among the wraps.
5. Tightly roll up each wrap, folding in the sides as you go.
6. Cut the wraps in half diagonally before serving, if desired.
7. Serve Greek chickpea and quinoa wraps immediately.

Nutrition Facts (per serving):

- Calories: 350
- Carbohydrates: 45g
- Protein: 10g
- Fat: 15g

80. Teriyaki Turkey and Vegetable Skewers

Prep.Time: 15 min

Cook Time: 10 min

Serving: 4

Beverage pairing: Jasmine Tea

Ingredients:

- 1 lb turkey breast, cut into cubes
- 2 cups mixed vegetables (such as bell peppers, onions, zucchini)
- 1/2 cup teriyaki sauce
- Wooden or metal skewers

Preparation:

1. If using wooden skewers, soak them in water for at least 30 minutes to prevent burning.
2. Preheat grill or grill pan to medium-high heat.
3. Thread turkey cubes and mixed vegetables onto skewers, alternating between turkey and vegetables.
4. Brush skewers with teriyaki sauce, coating them evenly.
5. Place skewers on the preheated grill or grill pan.
6. Grill skewers for 8-10 minutes, turning occasionally, until turkey is cooked through and vegetables are tender.
7. Remove skewers from the grill and let them rest for a few minutes before serving.
8. Serve teriyaki turkey and vegetable skewers hot.

Nutrition Facts (per serving, 2 skewers):

- Calories: 300
- Carbohydrates: 20g
- Protein: 25g
- Fat: 10g

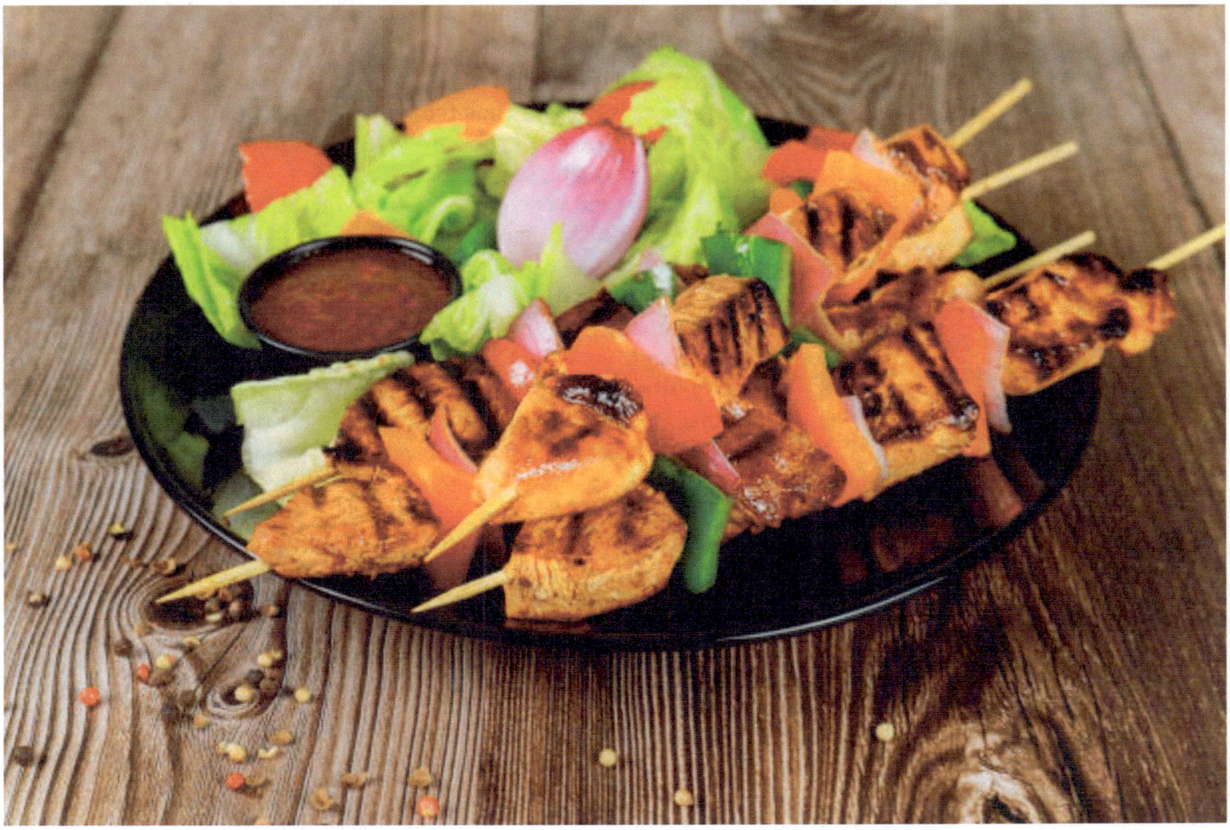

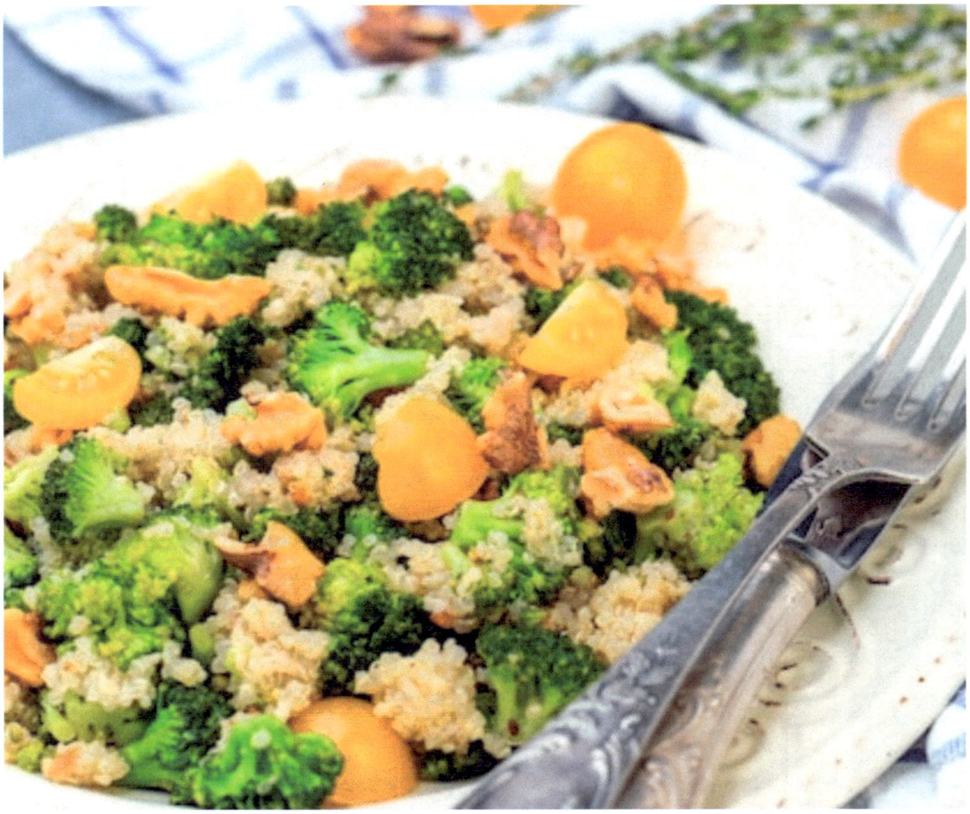

81. Turkey and Broccoli Cauliflower Fried Rice

Prep.Time: 15 min

Cook Time: 15 min

Serving: 4

Beverage pairing: Green Tea

Ingredients:

- 1 lb ground turkey
- 2 cups cauliflower rice
- 1 cup broccoli florets, chopped
- 1/2 cup carrots, diced
- 1/2 cup peas
- 2 cloves garlic, minced
- 2 tablespoons soy sauce or tamari
- 1 tablespoon sesame oil
- 1 tablespoon olive oil
- Salt and pepper to taste
- Green onions for garnish (optional)
- Sesame seeds for garnish (optional)

Preparation:

1. Heat olive oil in a large skillet or wok over medium-high heat.
2. Add ground turkey to the skillet and cook until browned, breaking it up into crumbles with a spatula.
3. Stir in minced garlic and cook for another minute until fragrant.
4. Add chopped broccoli, diced carrots, and peas to the skillet. Cook for 3-4 minutes until vegetables are tender-crisp.
5. Push the turkey and vegetable mixture to one side of the skillet. Add cauliflower rice to the empty side of the skillet.
6. Drizzle sesame oil and soy sauce over the cauliflower rice. Stir to combine with the turkey and vegetable mixture.
7. Cook for another 3-4 minutes, stirring occasionally, until cauliflower rice is heated through.
8. Season with salt and pepper to taste.
9. Garnish with chopped green onions and sesame seeds if desired.
10. Serve turkey and broccoli cauliflower fried rice hot.

Nutrition Facts (per serving):

- Calories: 300
- Carbohydrates: 15g
- Protein: 25g
- Fat: 15g

82. Caprese Chicken and Spinach Salad

Prep.Time: 10 min

Cook Time: 12 min

Serving: 2

Beverage pairing: Mint Water

Ingredients:

- 2 boneless, skinless chicken breasts
- Salt and pepper to taste
- 2 tablespoons olive oil
- 2 cups baby spinach leaves
- 1 cup cherry tomatoes, halved
- 1/2 cup fresh mozzarella balls, halved
- 2 tablespoons balsamic glaze
- Fresh basil leaves for garnish (optional)

Preparation:

1. Season chicken breasts with salt and pepper to taste.
2. Heat olive oil in a skillet over medium-high heat.
3. Add chicken breasts to the skillet and cook for 5-6 minutes per side, or until cooked through and no longer pink in the center.
4. Remove chicken from the skillet and let it rest for a few minutes before slicing.
5. In a large salad bowl, combine baby spinach leaves, halved cherry tomatoes, and halved fresh mozzarella balls.
6. Top the salad with sliced cooked chicken breasts.
7. Drizzle balsamic glaze over the salad.
8. Garnish with fresh basil leaves if desired.
9. Serve Caprese chicken and spinach salad immediately.

Nutrition Facts (per serving):

- Calories: 300
- Carbohydrates: 10g
- Protein: 30g
- Fat: 15g

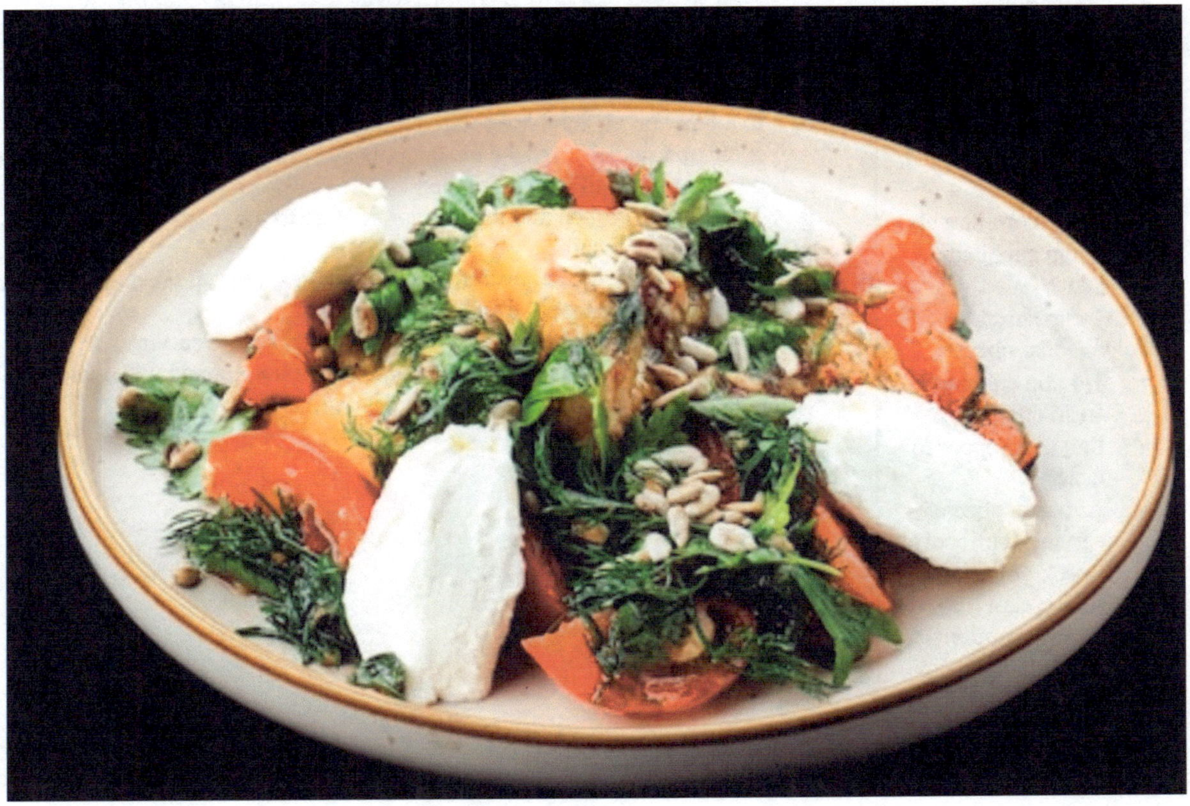

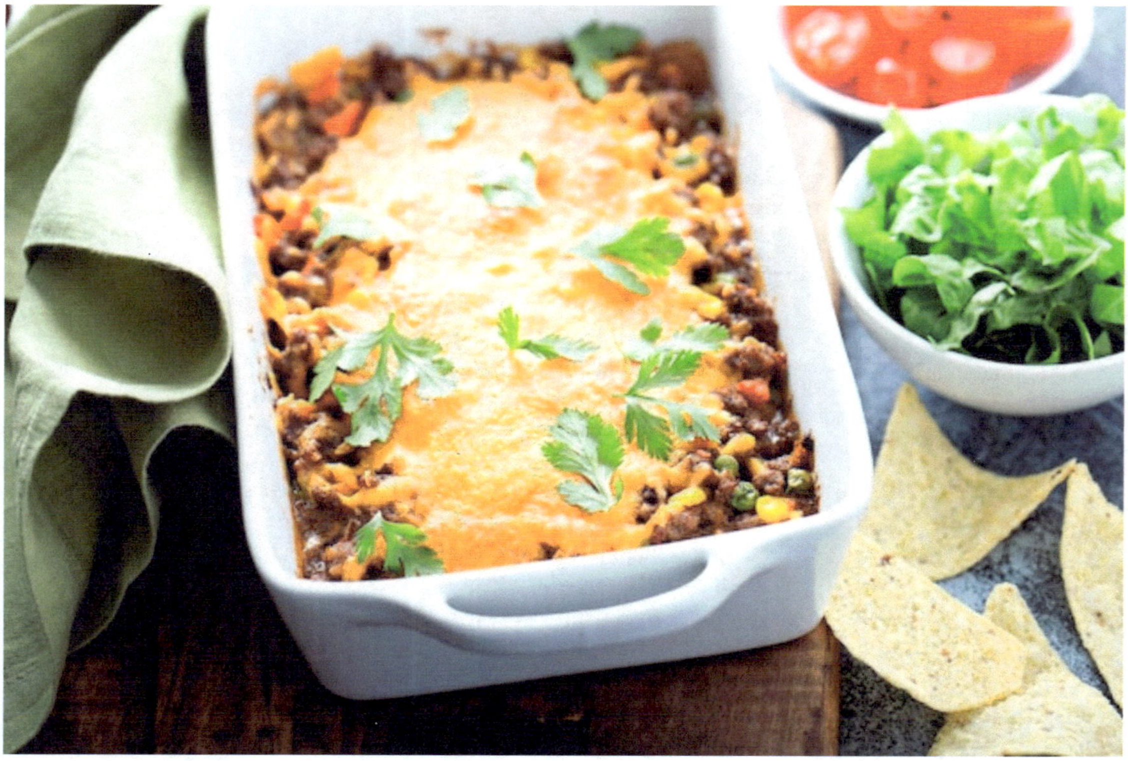

83. Quinoa and Black Bean Enchilada Bake

Prep.Time: 15 min

Cook Time: 25 min

Serving: 6

Beverage pairing: Green Tea

Ingredients:

- 1 cup quinoa, rinsed
- 2 cups vegetable broth
- 1 can (15 oz) black beans, drained and rinsed
- 1 cup corn kernels
- 1 cup enchilada sauce
- 1 cup shredded cheddar cheese
- 1/4 cup chopped fresh cilantro
- Salt and pepper to taste
- Avocado slices for serving (optional)
- Greek yogurt or sour cream for serving (optional)

Preparation:

1. Preheat oven to 375°F (190°C). Grease a 9x13-inch baking dish.
2. In a saucepan, combine quinoa and vegetable broth. Bring to a boil, then reduce heat to low, cover, and simmer for 15-20 minutes, or until quinoa is cooked and liquid is absorbed. Remove from heat and fluff with a fork.
3. In a large bowl, combine cooked quinoa, black beans, corn kernels, enchilada sauce, shredded cheddar cheese, chopped fresh cilantro, salt, and pepper. Mix until well combined.
4. Transfer the quinoa and black bean mixture to the prepared baking dish. Spread it out evenly.
5. Bake in the preheated oven for 20-25 minutes, or until the edges are bubbly and the cheese is melted and golden brown.
6. Remove from the oven and let it cool slightly before serving.
7. Serve quinoa and black bean enchilada bake hot, topped with avocado slices and Greek yogurt or sour cream if desired.

Nutrition Facts (per serving):

- Calories: 350
- Carbohydrates: 45g
- Protein: 15g
- Fat: 15g

84. Greek Yogurt Chicken and Cucumber Wrap

Prep.Time: 10 min

Cook Time: 0 min

Serving: 4

Beverage pairing: Herbal Tea

Ingredients:

- 4 whole wheat wraps or tortillas
- 2 cups cooked chicken breast, shredded or sliced
- 1 cup Greek yogurt
- 1 cucumber, thinly sliced
- 1/4 cup chopped fresh dill
- 2 tablespoons lemon juice
- Salt and pepper to taste
- Red onion slices for garnish (optional)

Preparation:

1. In a bowl, combine cooked chicken breast, Greek yogurt, chopped fresh dill, lemon juice, salt, and pepper. Mix until well combined.
2. Lay out the whole wheat wraps or tortillas on a flat surface.
3. Spread a layer of the Greek yogurt chicken mixture onto each wrap.
4. Top the chicken mixture with thinly sliced cucumber slices.
5. Roll up each wrap tightly, folding in the sides as you go.
6. Cut the wraps in half diagonally before serving, if desired.
7. Garnish with red onion slices if desired.
8. Serve Greek yogurt chicken and cucumber wraps immediately.

Nutrition Facts (per serving):

- Calories: 300
- Carbohydrates: 25g
- Protein: 30g
- Fat: 10g

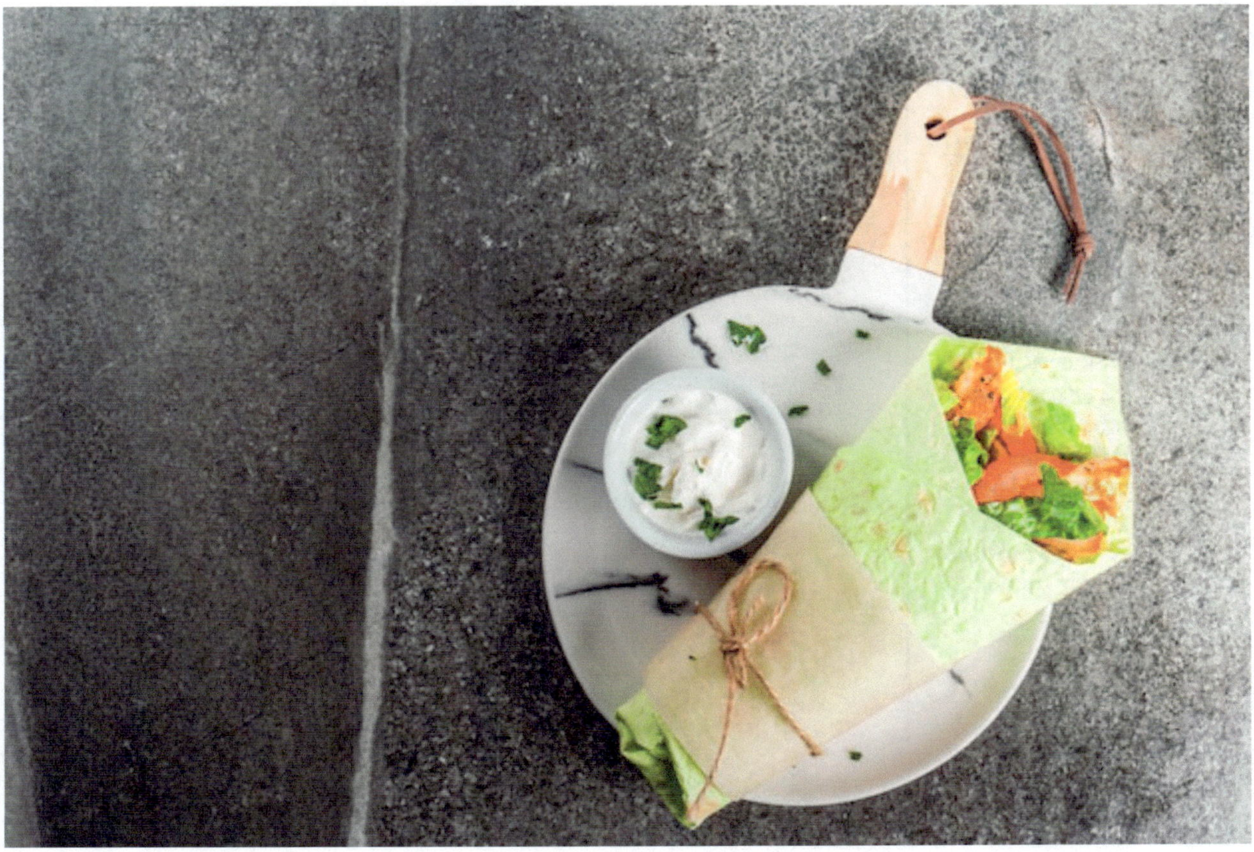

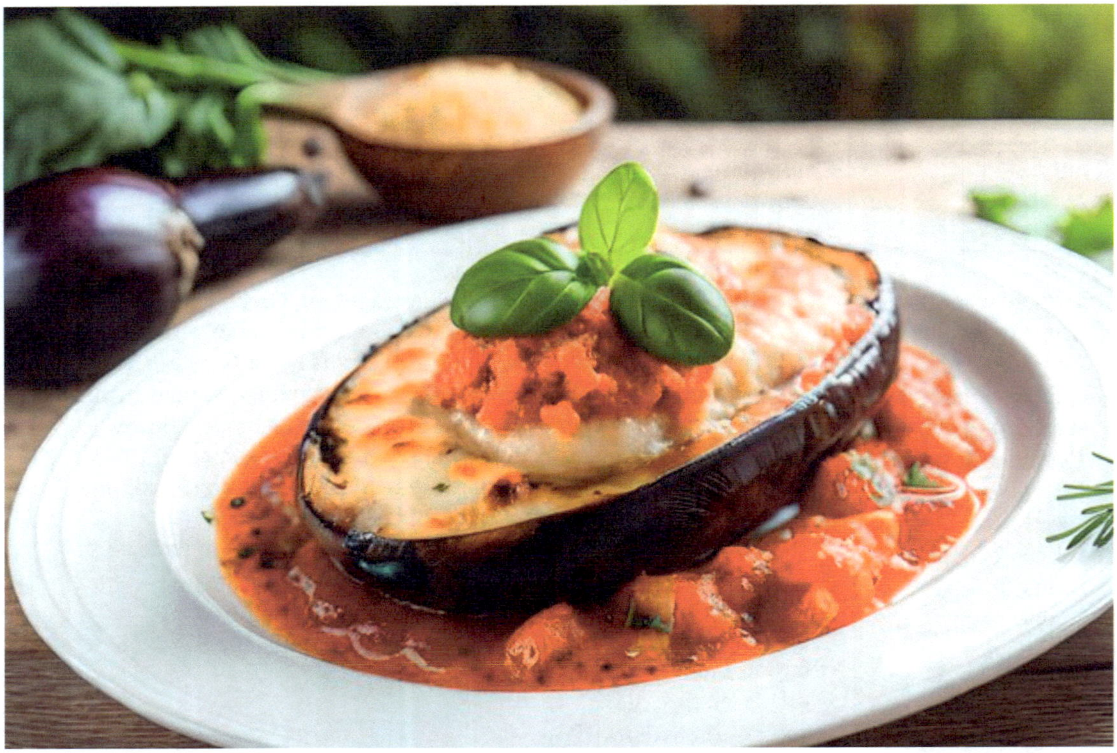

85. Squash Boat with Tomato Basil Sauce

Prep.Time: 10 min

Cook Time: 20 min

Serving: 4

Beverage pairing: Mint Water

Ingredients:

- 4 Squash boat
- Salt and pepper to taste
- 2 tablespoons olive oil
- 2 cloves garlic, minced
- 1 can (14.5 oz) diced tomatoes
- 1/4 cup chopped fresh basil
- 1/2 teaspoon dried oregano
- 1/4 teaspoon crushed red pepper flakes (optional)
- Lemon wedges for serving (optional)

Preparation:

1. Preheat oven to 400°F (200°C). Grease a baking dish with olive oil.
2. Season squash fillets with salt and pepper to taste.
3. Heat olive oil in a skillet over medium heat.
4. Add minced garlic to the skillet and cook for 1 minute until fragrant.
5. Stir in diced tomatoes, chopped fresh basil, dried oregano, and crushed red pepper flakes (if using). Cook for 5-7 minutes, stirring occasionally, until the sauce thickens slightly.
6. Place seasoned squash boat in the prepared baking dish.
7. Pour the tomato basil sauce over the squash fillets, covering them evenly.
8. Bake in the preheated oven for 15-20 minutes, or until the squash is cooked through and flakes easily with a fork.
9. Remove from the oven and let it cool slightly before serving.
10. Serve squash boat with tomato basil sauce hot, with lemon wedges if desired.

Nutrition Facts (per serving):

- Calories: 250
- Carbohydrates: 5g
- Protein: 30g
- Fat: 10g

86. Lentil and Vegetable Stew with Sweet Potatoes

Prep.Time: 15 min

Cook Time: 45 min

Serving: 6

Beverage pairing: Herbal Tea

Ingredients:

- 1 cup green lentils, rinsed
- 4 cups vegetable broth
- 2 sweet potatoes, peeled and diced
- 1 onion, diced
- 2 carrots, diced
- 2 celery stalks, diced
- 2 cloves garlic, minced
- 1 can (14.5 oz) diced tomatoes
- 1 teaspoon dried thyme
- 1 teaspoon dried rosemary
- Salt and pepper to taste
- Chopped fresh parsley for garnish (optional)

Preparation:

1. In a large pot, combine green lentils and vegetable broth. Bring to a boil, then reduce heat to low, cover, and simmer for 20 minutes.
2. Add diced sweet potatoes, diced onion, diced carrots, diced celery, minced garlic, diced tomatoes (with juices), dried thyme, and dried rosemary to the pot.
3. Stir to combine and bring the stew back to a simmer.
4. Cook for an additional 20-25 minutes, or until the lentils and vegetables are tender.
5. Season with salt and pepper to taste.
6. Remove from heat and let the stew cool slightly before serving.
7. Garnish with chopped fresh parsley if desired.
8. Serve lentil and vegetable stew hot.

Nutrition Facts (per serving):

- Calories: 300
- Carbohydrates: 55g
- Protein: 15g
- Fat: 5g

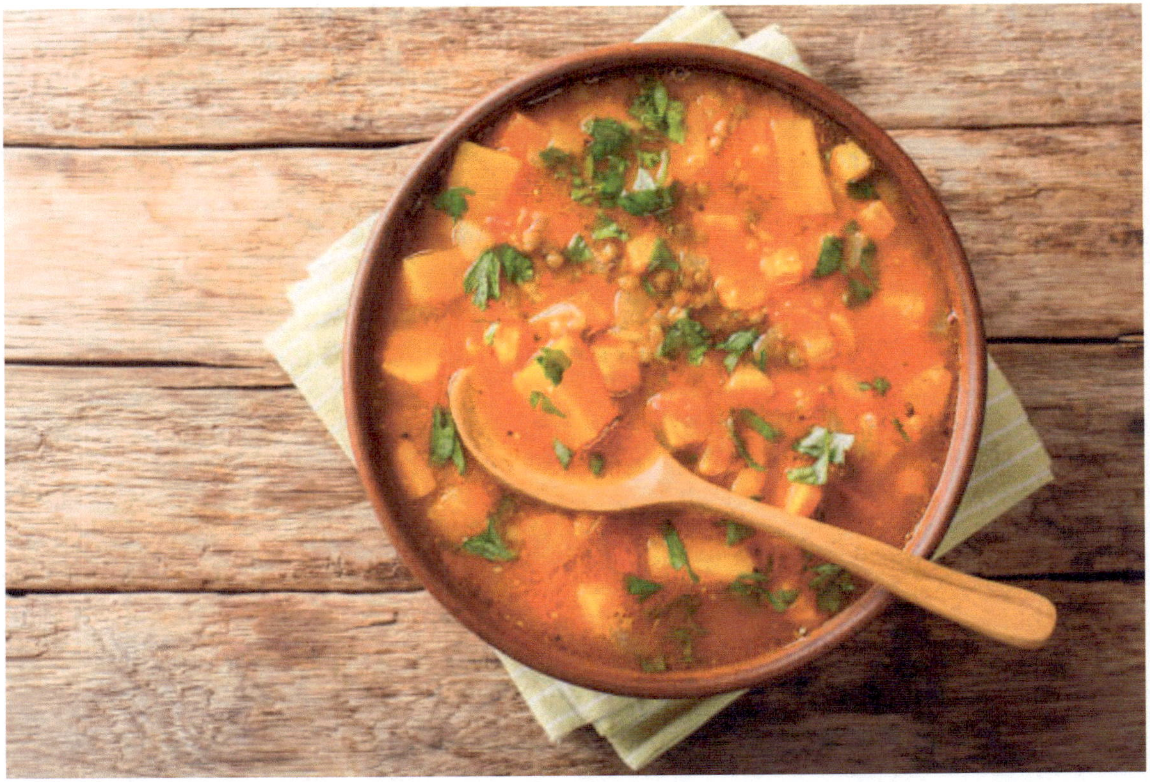

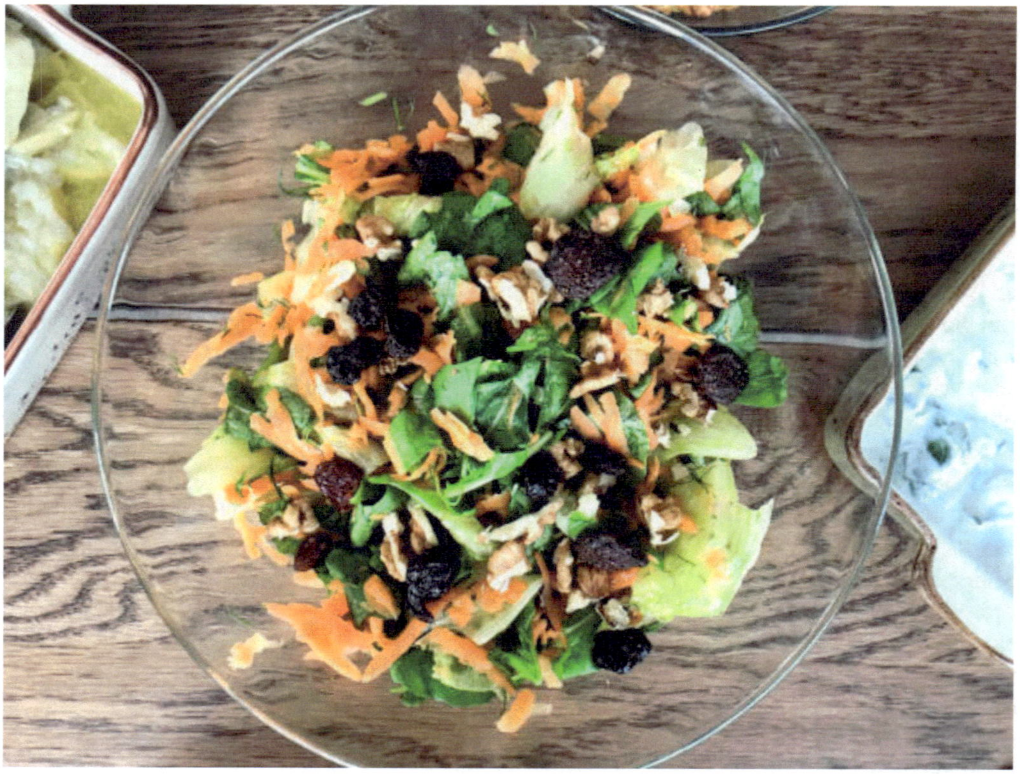

87. Turkey and Cranberry Spinach Salad

Prep.Time: 10 min

Cook Time: 0 min

Serving: 4

Beverage pairing: Mint Water

Ingredients:

- 2 cups cooked turkey breast, shredded or sliced
- 4 cups baby spinach leaves
- 1/2 cup dried cranberries
- 1/4 cup chopped pecans
- 1/4 cup crumbled feta cheese
- Balsamic vinaigrette for dressing

Preparation:

1. In a large salad bowl, combine cooked turkey breast, baby spinach leaves, dried cranberries, chopped pecans, and crumbled feta cheese.
2. Drizzle balsamic vinaigrette over the salad.
3. Toss gently to coat the ingredients evenly with the dressing.
4. Serve turkey and cranberry spinach salad immediately.

Nutrition Facts (per serving):

- Calories: 300
- Carbohydrates: 20g
- Protein: 25g
- Fat: 15g

88. Shrimp and Avocado Zoodle Bowl

Prep.Time: 15 min

Cook Time: 10 min

Serving: 4

Beverage pairing: Mint Water

Ingredients:

- 1 lb shrimp, peeled and deveined
- Salt and pepper to taste
- 2 tablespoons olive oil
- 2 zucchinis, spiralized into noodles
- 1 avocado, diced
- 1 cup cherry tomatoes, halved
- 1/4 cup chopped fresh cilantro
- Juice of 1 lime
- Red pepper flakes for garnish (optional)

Preparation:

1. Season shrimp with salt and pepper to taste.
2. Heat olive oil in a large skillet over medium-high heat.
3. Add shrimp to the skillet and cook for 2-3 minutes per side, or until pink and cooked through.
4. Remove shrimp from the skillet and set aside.
5. In the same skillet, add spiralized zucchini noodles. Cook for 2-3 minutes until tender but still crisp.
6. Transfer cooked zucchini noodles to serving bowls.
7. Top the zucchini noodles with cooked shrimp, diced avocado, halved cherry tomatoes, chopped fresh cilantro, and lime juice.
8. Garnish with red pepper flakes if desired.
9. Serve shrimp and avocado zoodle bowls immediately.

Nutrition Facts (per serving):

- Calories: 300
- Carbohydrates: 15g
- Protein: 25g
- Fat: 15g

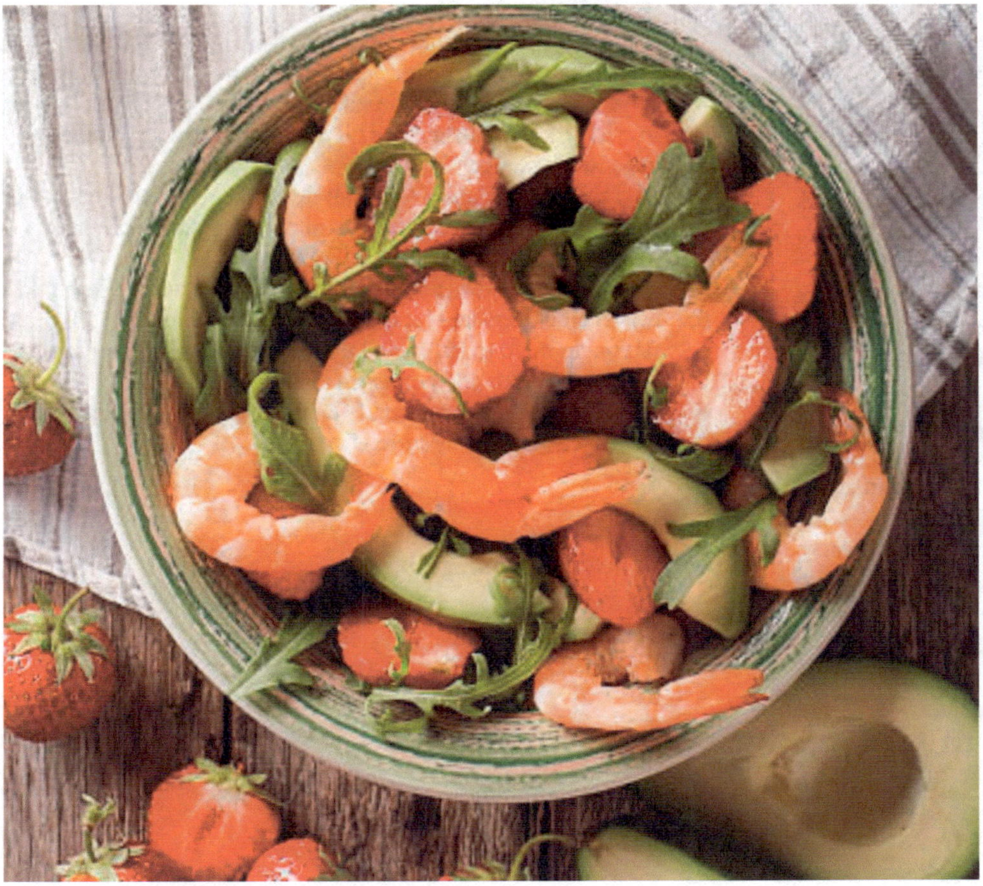

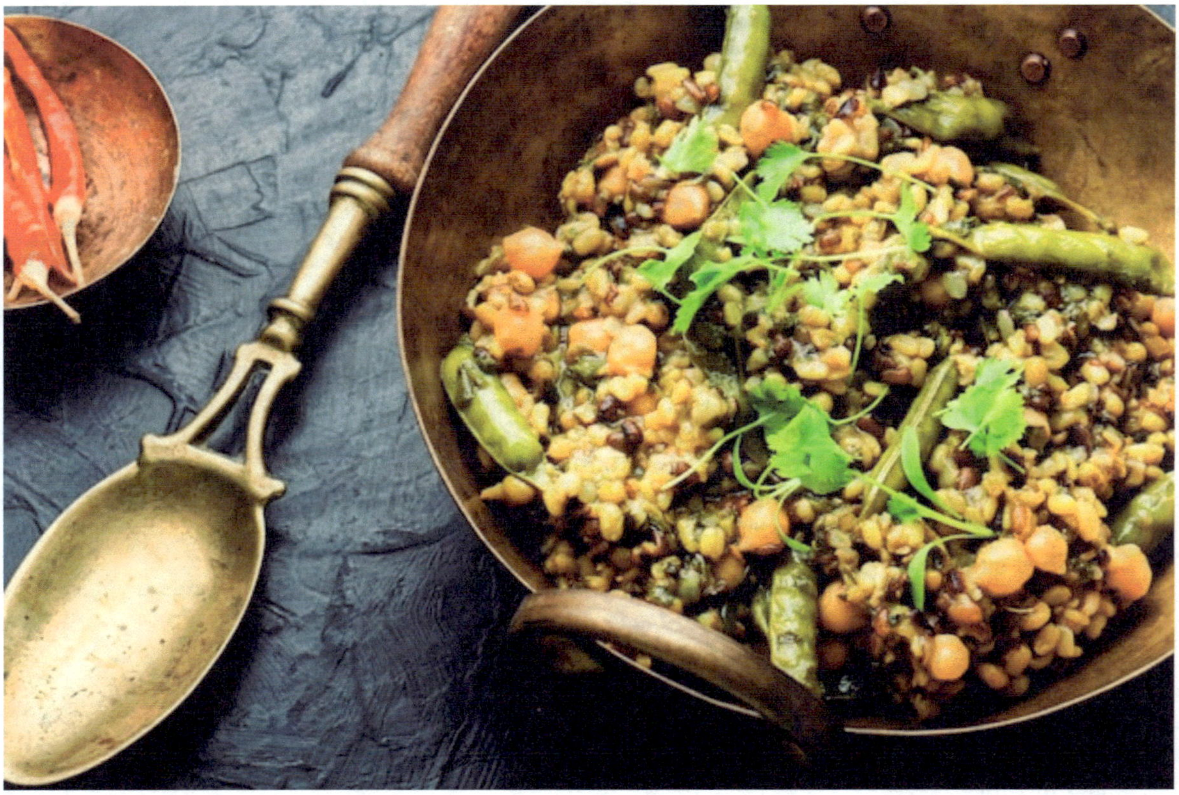

89. Chickpea and Vegetable Curry with Quinoa

Prep.Time: 15 min

Cook Time: 25 min

Serving: 4

Beverage pairing: Chai

Ingredients:

- 1 cup quinoa, rinsed
- 2 cups vegetable broth
- 1 can (15 oz) chickpeas, drained and rinsed
- 2 cups mixed vegetables (such as bell peppers, carrots, peas)
- 1 onion, diced
- 2 cloves garlic, minced
- 1 tablespoon curry powder
- 1 teaspoon ground cumin
- 1 teaspoon ground coriander
- 1 can (14 oz) diced tomatoes
- 1 can (14 oz) coconut milk

Preparation:

1. In a saucepan, combine quinoa and vegetable broth. Bring to a boil, then reduce heat to low, cover, and simmer for 15-20 minutes, or until quinoa is cooked and liquid is absorbed. Remove from heat and fluff with a fork.
2. In a large skillet, heat olive oil over medium heat. Add diced onion and minced garlic. Sauté until onions are translucent.
3. Add mixed vegetables to the skillet and cook until slightly softened.
4. Stir in curry powder, ground cumin, and ground coriander. Cook for another minute until fragrant.
5. Add diced tomatoes and coconut milk to the skillet. Bring to a simmer.
6. Stir in chickpeas and let the mixture simmer for 10-15 minutes, allowing the flavors to meld together and the vegetables to become tender.
7. Season with salt and pepper to taste.
8. Serve chickpea and vegetable curry over cooked quinoa.
9. Garnish with fresh cilantro if desired.

Nutrition Facts (per serving):

- Calories: 400
- Carbohydrates: 50g
- Protein: 15g
- Fat: 18g

90. Turkey and Pesto Zucchini Noodle Bowl

Prep.Time: 15 min

Cook Time: 15 min

Serving: 4

Beverage pairing: Lemonade

Ingredients:

- 2 large zucchinis, spiralized into noodles
- 1 lb ground turkey
- 2 tablespoons olive oil
- 1/4 cup pesto sauce
- 1 cup cherry tomatoes, halved
- 1/4 cup grated Parmesan cheese
- Salt and pepper to taste
- Fresh basil leaves for garnish (optional)

Preparation:

1. Heat olive oil in a large skillet over medium heat.
2. Add ground turkey to the skillet and cook until browned, breaking it up into crumbles with a spatula.
3. Stir in pesto sauce and cherry tomatoes. Cook for another 3-4 minutes until tomatoes are softened.
4. Add spiralized zucchini noodles to the skillet. Toss to combine with the turkey and pesto mixture.
5. Cook for 2-3 minutes until zucchini noodles are heated through but still slightly crisp.
6. Season with salt and pepper to taste.
7. Divide the turkey and pesto zucchini noodles into serving bowls.
8. Sprinkle grated Parmesan cheese over each bowl.
9. Garnish with fresh basil leaves if desired.
10. Serve turkey and pesto zucchini noodle bowls immediately.

Nutrition Facts (per serving):

- Calories: 350
- Carbohydrates: 10g
- Protein: 25g
- Fat: 25g

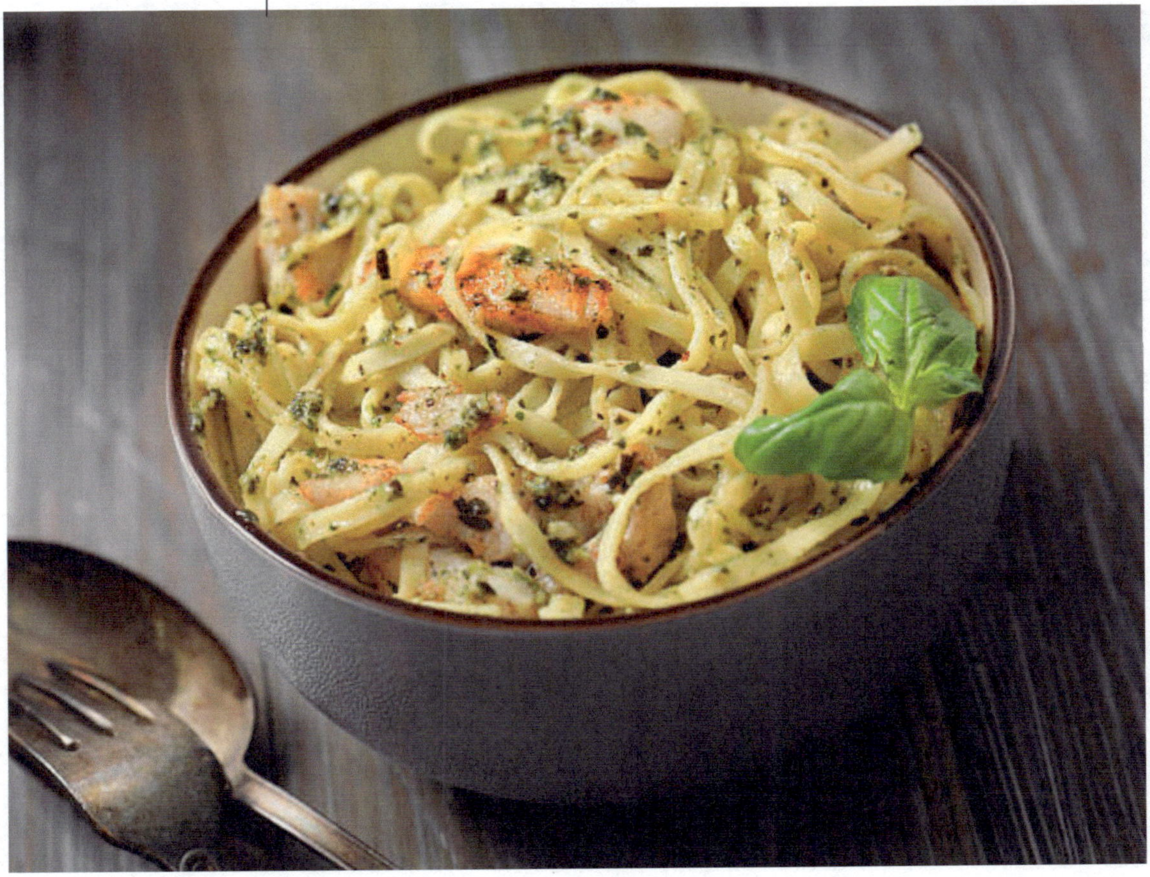

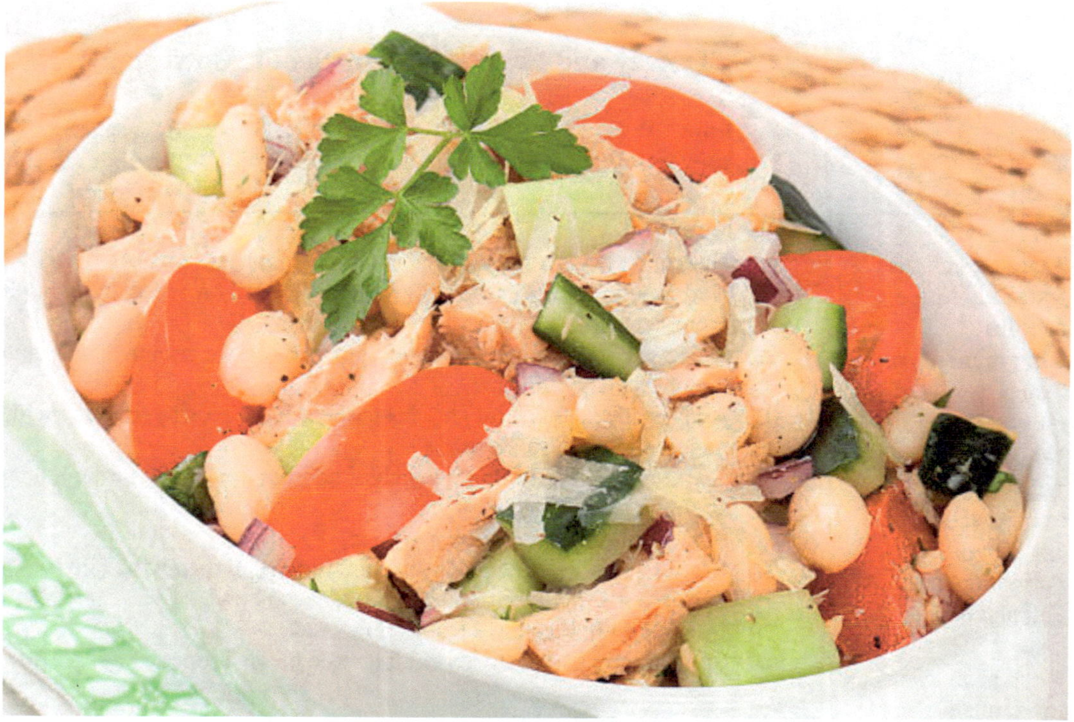

91. Mediterranean Tuna and White Bean Salad

Prep.Time: 10 min

Cook Time: 0 min

Serving: 4

Beverage pairing: Lemonade

Ingredients:

- 2 cans (5 oz each) tuna in water, drained
- 1 can (15 oz) cannellini beans, drained and rinsed
- 1 cucumber, diced
- 1 cup cherry tomatoes, halved
- 1/4 cup sliced Kalamata olives
- 1/4 cup chopped fresh parsley
- Juice of 1 lemon
- 2 tablespoons extra-virgin olive oil
- Salt and pepper to taste
- Crumbled feta cheese for garnish (optional)

Preparation:

1. In a large salad bowl, combine drained tuna, cannellini beans, diced cucumber, halved cherry tomatoes, sliced Kalamata olives, and chopped fresh parsley.
2. Drizzle lemon juice and extra-virgin olive oil over the salad.
3. Toss gently to combine all the ingredients.
4. Season with salt and pepper to taste.
5. Garnish with crumbled feta cheese if desired.
6. Serve Mediterranean tuna and white bean salad immediately.

Nutrition Facts (per serving):

- Calories: 300
- Carbohydrates: 25g
- Protein: 30g
- Fat: 10g

92. Chicken and Vegetable Burrito

Prep.Time: 20 min

Cook Time: 25 min

Serving: 4

Beverage pairing: Lemonade

Ingredients:

- 1 cup quinoa, rinsed
- 2 cups chicken broth
- 1 lb boneless, skinless chicken breasts
- 1 tablespoon olive oil
- 1 onion, diced
- 2 cloves garlic, minced
- 1 bell pepper, diced
- 1 cup corn kernels
- 1 can (15 oz) black beans, drained and rinsed
- 1 teaspoon chili powder
- 1 teaspoon ground cumin

Preparation:

1. In a saucepan, combine quinoa and chicken broth. Bring to a boil, then reduce heat to low, cover, and simmer for 15-20 minutes, or until quinoa is cooked and liquid is absorbed. Remove from heat and fluff with a fork.
2. Season chicken breasts with chili powder, ground cumin, salt, and pepper.
3. Heat olive oil in a skillet over medium-high heat. Add chicken breasts and cook for 5-6 minutes per side, or until cooked through and no longer pink in the center. Remove from the skillet and let them rest for a few minutes before slicing.
4. In the same skillet, add diced onion and minced garlic. Sauté until onions are translucent.
5. Add diced bell pepper and corn kernels to the skillet. Cook for 3-4 minutes until vegetables are tender.
6. Stir in black beans and cooked quinoa. Cook for another 2-3 minutes to heat through. Divide the quinoa and vegetable mixture into serving bowls.
7. Top each bowl with sliced cooked chicken breasts.
8. Serve chicken and vegetable burrito immediately, garnished with avocado slices, Greek yogurt or sour cream, and fresh cilantro if desired.

Nutrition Facts (per serving):

- Calories: 400
- Carbohydrates: 40g
- Protein: 30g
- Fat: 15g

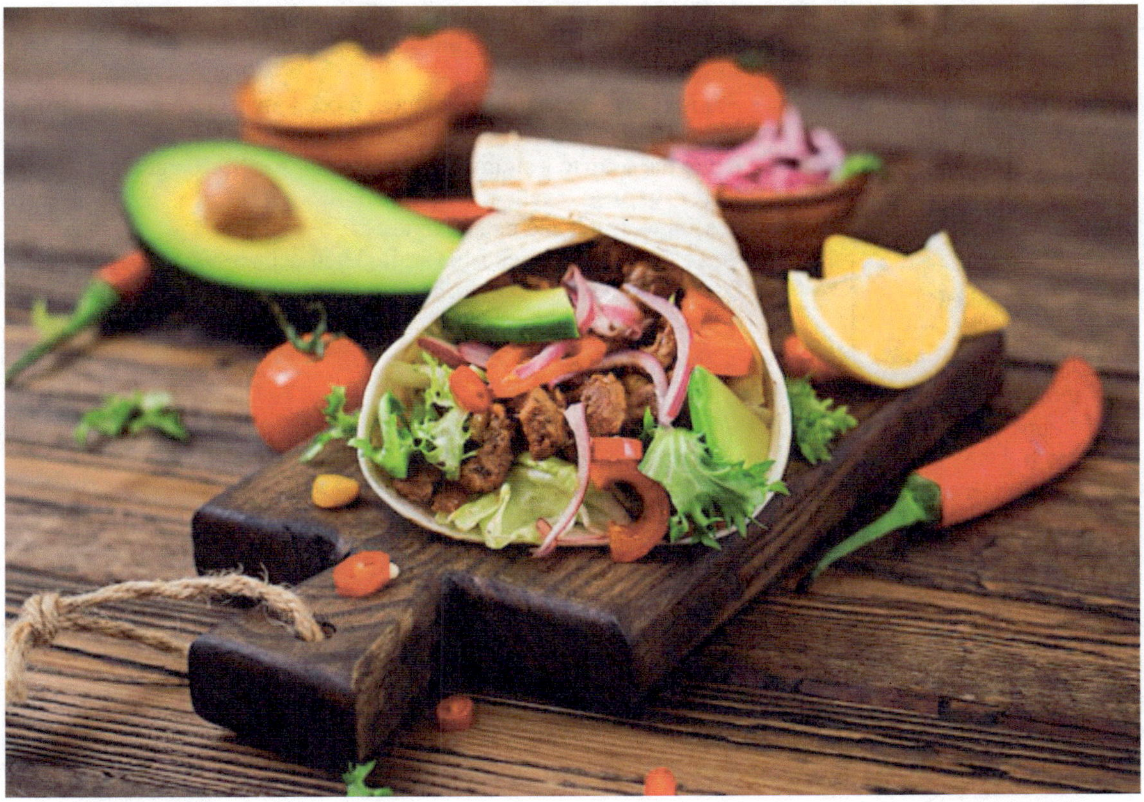

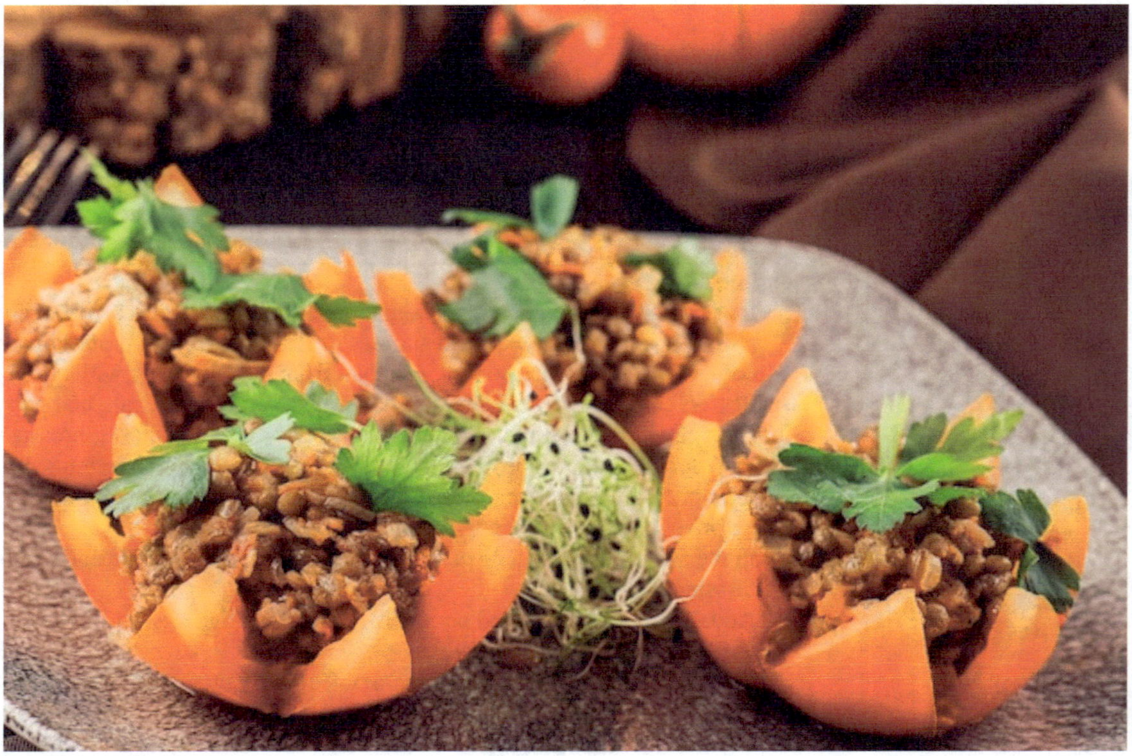

93. Quinoa and Black Bean Stuffed Bell Pepper

Prep.Time: 10 min

Cook Time: 25 min

Serving: 4

Beverage pairing: Veges Broth

Ingredients:

- 1 tablespoon olive oil
- 1 onion, diced
- 2 cloves garlic, minced
- 2 bell peppers, diced
- 1 can (15 oz) black beans, drained and rinsed
- 1 cup cooked quinoa
- 1 can (14 oz) diced tomatoes
- 4 cups vegetable broth
- 1 teaspoon cumin
- 1 teaspoon chili powder

Preparation:

1. Heat olive oil in a large pot over medium heat. Add diced onion and minced garlic. Sauté until onions are translucent.
2. Add diced bell peppers to the pot and cook for 3-4 minutes until slightly softened.
3. Stir in black beans, cooked quinoa, diced tomatoes, vegetable broth, cumin, and chili powder.
4. Bring the soup to a simmer and let it cook for 15-20 minutes, allowing the flavors to meld together.
5. Season with salt and pepper to taste.
6. Serve quinoa and black bean stuffed bell pepper hot.
7. Garnish with fresh cilantro, avocado slices, and Greek yogurt or sour cream if desired.

Nutrition Facts (per serving):

- Calories: 250
- Carbohydrates: 35g
- Protein: 10g
- Fat: 7g

94. Grilled Lemon Herb Turkey Skewers

Prep.Time: 10 min

Cook Time: 10 min

Serving: 4

Beverage pairing: Lemonade

Ingredients:

- 1 lb turkey breast, cut into cubes
- 2 tablespoons olive oil
- 2 cloves garlic, minced
- Zest and juice of 1 lemon
- 1 tablespoon chopped fresh rosemary
- 1 tablespoon chopped fresh thyme
- Salt and pepper to taste
- Wooden or metal skewers

Preparation:

1. In a bowl, combine olive oil, minced garlic, lemon zest, lemon juice, chopped fresh rosemary, chopped fresh thyme, salt, and pepper.
2. Add turkey cubes to the bowl and toss to coat them evenly with the marinade. Cover and refrigerate for at least 30 minutes, or up to 2 hours.
3. Preheat grill or grill pan to medium-high heat.
4. Thread marinated turkey cubes onto skewers.
5. Grill skewers for 8-10 minutes, turning occasionally, until turkey is cooked through and lightly charred on the outside.
6. Remove skewers from the grill and let them rest for a few minutes before serving.
7. Serve grilled lemon herb turkey skewers hot.

Nutrition Facts (per serving, 2 skewers):

- Calories: 300
- Carbohydrates: 2g
- Protein: 40g
- Fat: 15g

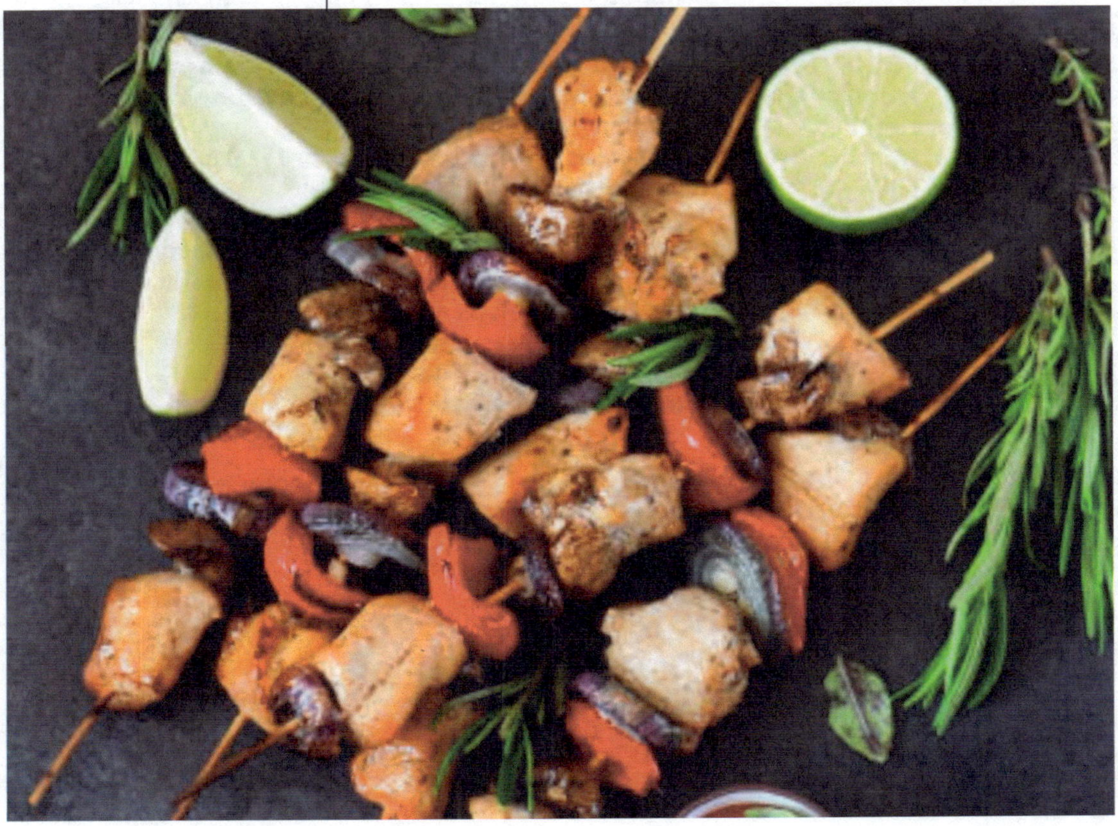

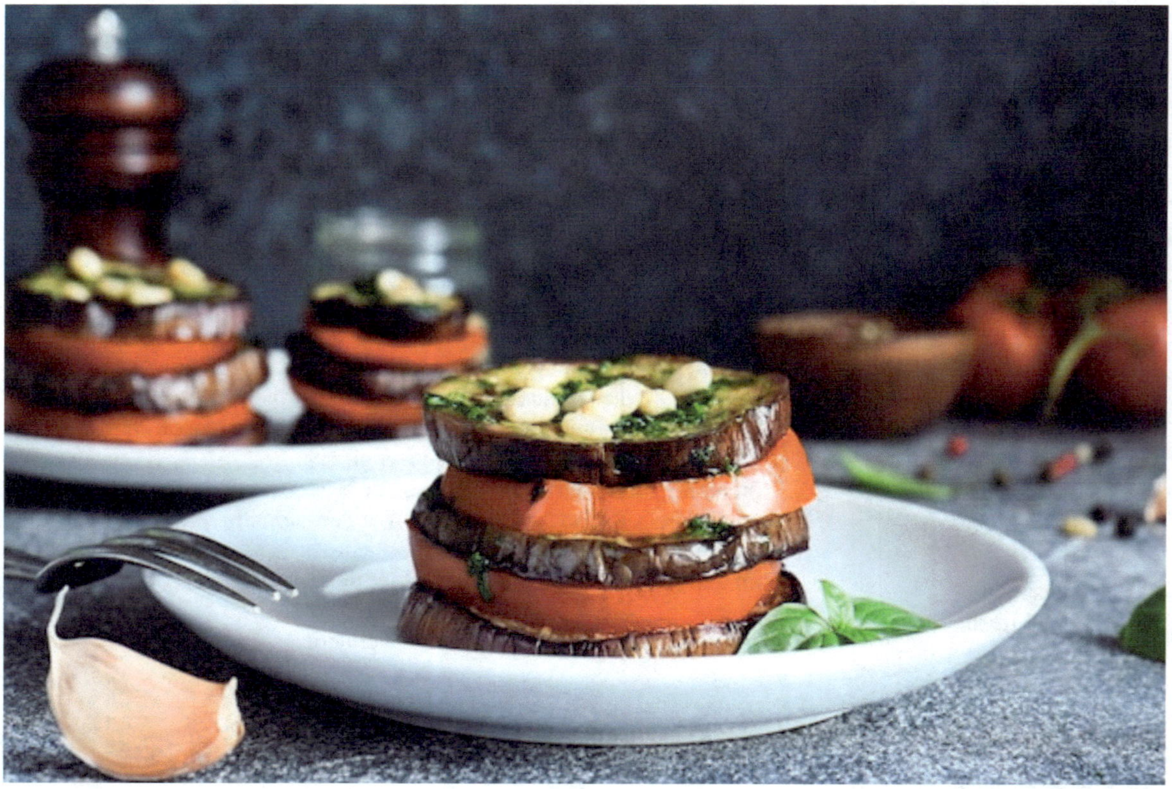

95. Caprese Eggplant and Spinach Stack

Prep.Time:	Cook Time:	Serving:	Beverage pairing:
10 min	20 min	2	Cranberry Juice

Ingredients:

- 1 large eggplant, sliced into rounds
- 2 tablespoons olive oil
- Salt and pepper to taste
- 1 cup cherry tomatoes, halved
- 1 cup fresh mozzarella cheese, sliced
- 1 cup baby spinach leaves
- Balsamic glaze for drizzling
- Fresh basil leaves for garnish (optional)

Preparation:

1. Preheat oven to 400°F (200°C). Line a baking sheet with parchment paper.
2. Place eggplant rounds on the prepared baking sheet. Brush both sides with olive oil and season with salt and pepper.
3. Roast eggplant rounds in the preheated oven for 15-20 minutes, flipping halfway through, until tender and lightly golden.
4. Remove eggplant rounds from the oven and let them cool slightly.
5. To assemble the stacks, layer one eggplant round with cherry tomato halves, fresh mozzarella slices, and baby spinach leaves. Repeat with another eggplant round and another layer of toppings.
6. Drizzle balsamic glaze over each stack.
7. Garnish with fresh basil leaves if desired.
8. Serve caprese eggplant and spinach stacks warm.

Nutrition Facts (per serving):

- Calories: 250
- Carbohydrates: 10g
- Protein: 10g
- Fat: 20g

96. Baked Salmon with Cucumber Dill Salad

Prep.Time: 10 min

Cook Time: 15 min

Serving: 4

Beverage pairing: Lemonade

Ingredients:

- 4 salmon fillets
- Salt and pepper to taste
- 2 tablespoons olive oil
- 1 cucumber, thinly sliced
- 1/4 cup chopped fresh dill
- 1/4 cup Greek yogurt
- 1 tablespoon lemon juice
- 1 teaspoon Dijon mustard
- Salt and pepper to taste

Preparation:

1. Preheat oven to 400°F (200°C). Line a baking sheet with parchment paper.
2. Place salmon fillets on the prepared baking sheet. Season with salt and pepper, and drizzle with olive oil.
3. Bake salmon in the preheated oven for 12-15 minutes, or until fish flakes easily with a fork.
4. In a bowl, combine thinly sliced cucumber, chopped fresh dill, Greek yogurt, lemon juice, Dijon mustard, salt, and pepper. Toss to coat the cucumber slices evenly.
5. Serve baked salmon hot, topped with cucumber dill salad.

Nutrition Facts (per serving):

- Calories: 300
- Carbohydrates: 5g
- Protein: 30g
- Fat: 18g

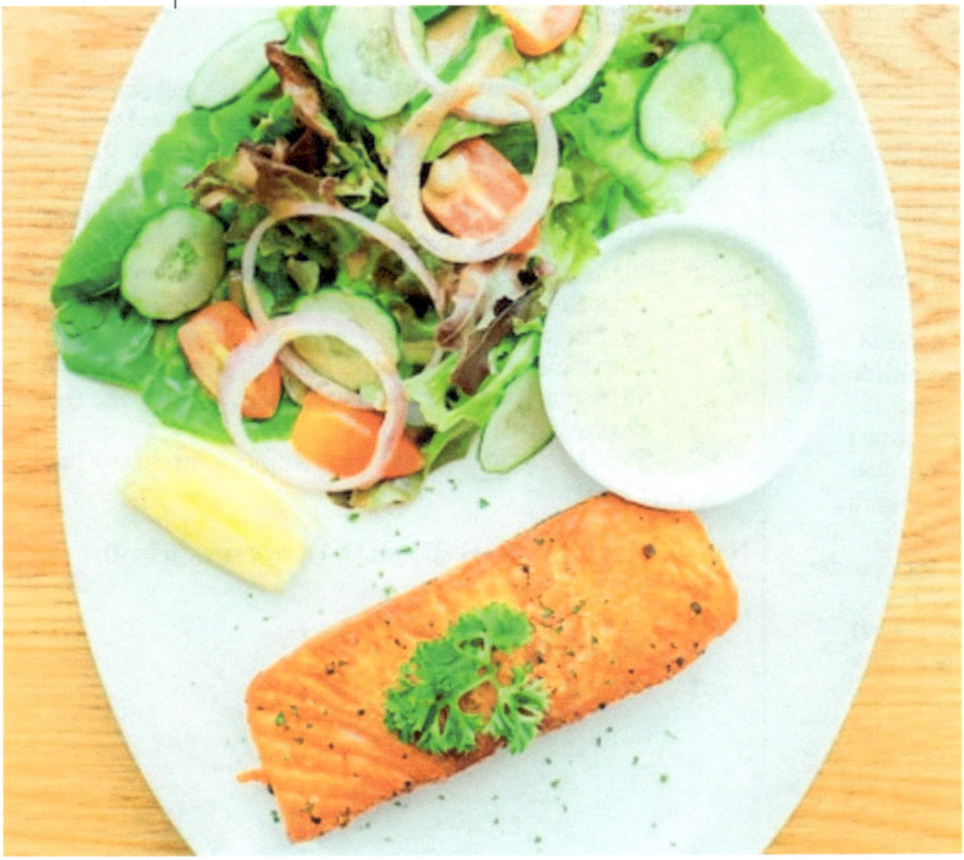

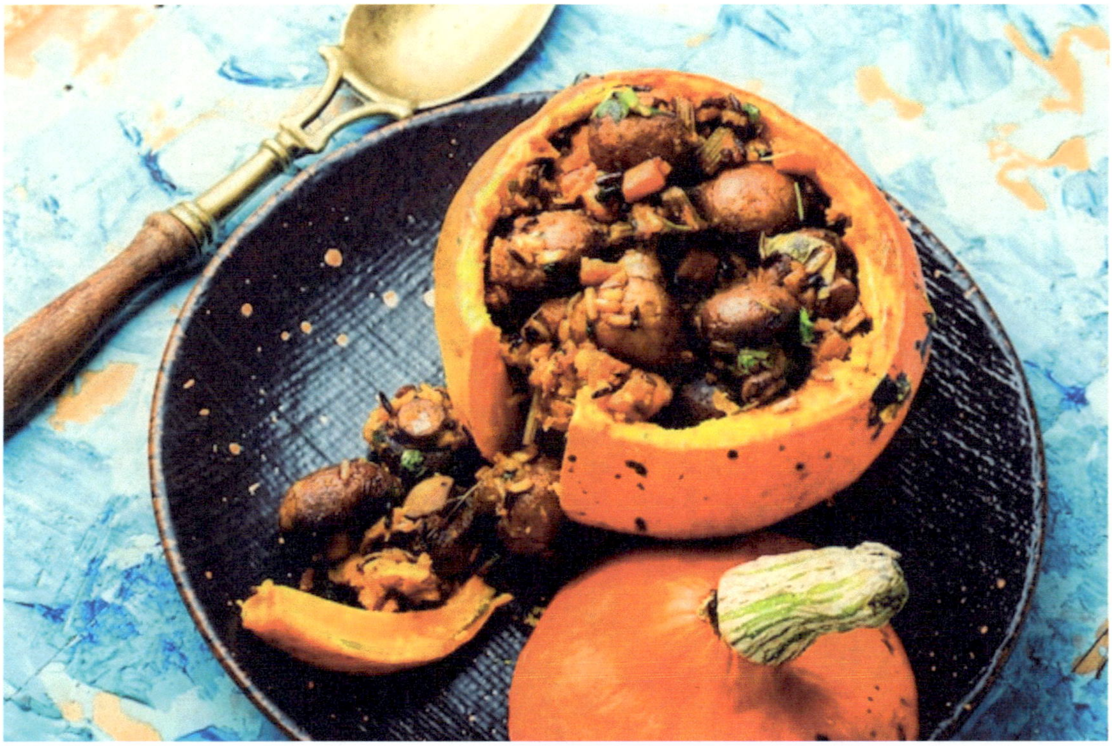

97. Lentil and Vegetable Curry Stuffed Acorn Squash

Prep.Time: 15 min

Cook Time: 30 min

Serving: 4

Beverage pairing: Tea

Ingredients:

- 2 acorn squash, halved and seeds removed
- 1 tablespoon olive oil
- Salt and pepper to taste
- 1 cup cooked lentils
- 1 cup mixed vegetables (such as bell peppers, carrots, peas)
- 1 onion, diced
- 2 cloves garlic, minced
- 1 tablespoon curry powder
- 1 can (14 oz) coconut milk

Preparation:

1. Preheat oven to 400°F (200°C).
2. Drizzle olive oil over halved acorn squash and season with salt and pepper. Place them cut side down on a baking sheet lined with parchment paper.
3. Roast acorn squash in the preheated oven for 25-30 minutes, or until tender.
4. In the meantime, heat olive oil in a skillet over medium heat. Add diced onion and minced garlic. Sauté until onions are translucent. Add mixed vegetables to the skillet and cook until slightly softened.
5. Stir in cooked lentils, curry powder, and coconut milk. Bring to a simmer and let the mixture cook for 5-7 minutes, allowing the flavors to meld together. Season with salt and pepper to taste.
6. Once the acorn squash halves are cooked, remove them from the oven and fill each half with lentil and vegetable curry mixture. Garnish with fresh cilantro if desired.
7. Serve lentil and vegetable curry stuffed acorn squash hot.

Nutrition Facts (per serving, 1 stuffed acorn squash half):

- Calories: 300
- Carbohydrates: 30g
- Protein: 10g
- Fat: 15g

98. Turkey and Avocado Caesar Salad

Prep.Time: 10 min | **Cook Time:** 0 min | **Serving:** 4 | **Beverage pairing:** Lemonade

Ingredients:

- 1 lb turkey breast, cooked and sliced
- 1 head romaine lettuce, chopped
- 1 avocado, sliced
- 1/2 cup cherry tomatoes, halved
- 1/4 cup grated Parmesan cheese
- Caesar dressing (store-bought or homemade)
- Salt and pepper to taste
- Croutons for garnish (optional)

Preparation:

1. In a large salad bowl, combine chopped romaine lettuce, sliced avocado, halved cherry tomatoes, and grated Parmesan cheese.
2. Add cooked and sliced turkey breast to the salad bowl.
3. Drizzle Caesar dressing over the salad, tossing to coat all the ingredients evenly.
4. Season with salt and pepper to taste.
5. Garnish with croutons if desired.
6. Serve turkey and avocado Caesar salad immediately.

Nutrition Facts (per serving):

- Calories: 350
- Carbohydrates: 15g
- Protein: 30g
- Fat: 20g

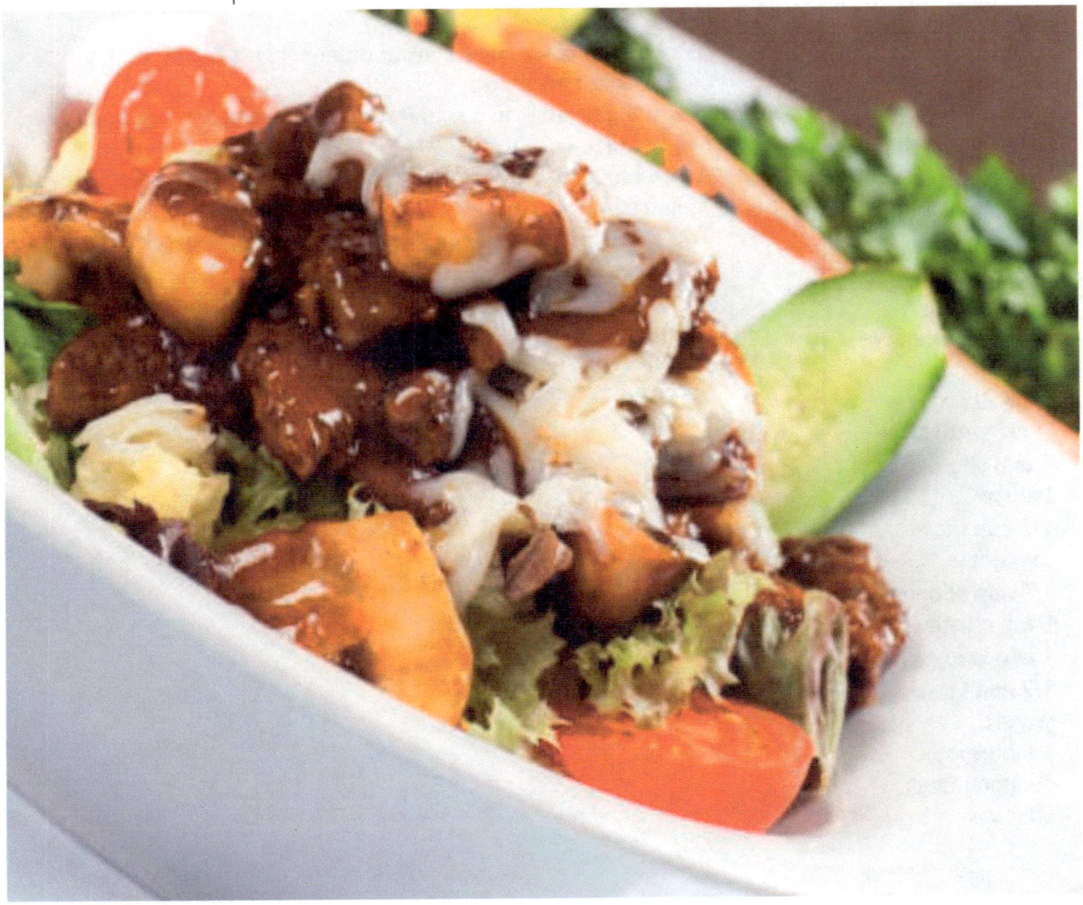

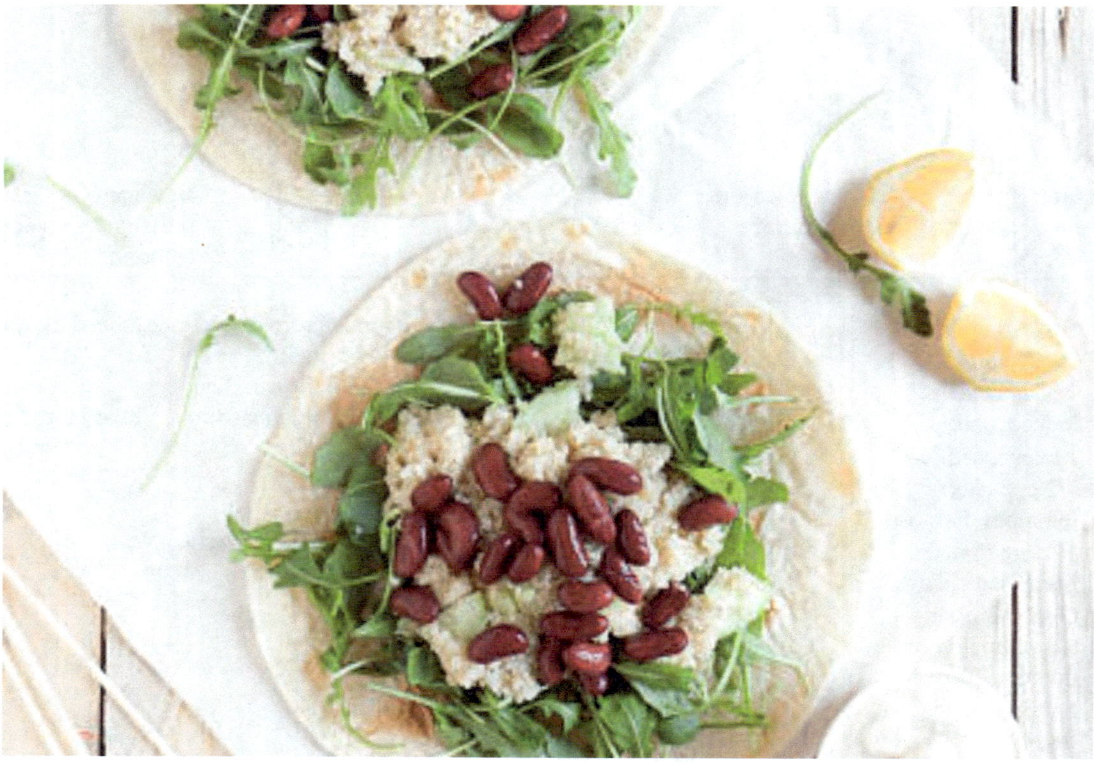

99. Quinoa and Black Bean Tacos with Greek Yogurt Sauce

Prep.Time:	Cook Time:	Serving:	Beverage pairing:
15 min	0 min	4	Green Tea

Ingredients:

- 1 cup cooked quinoa
- 1 can (15 oz) black beans, drained and rinsed
- 1 teaspoon chili powder
- 1/2 teaspoon ground cumin
- Salt and pepper to taste
- 8 small corn or flour tortillas
- 1 cup shredded lettuce
- 1/2 cup diced tomatoes
- 1/4 cup chopped fresh cilantro
- 1 avocado, sliced
- 1/2 cup Greek yogurt
- 1 tablespoon chopped fresh cilantro

Preparation:

1. In a bowl, mix together cooked quinoa, black beans, chili powder, ground cumin, salt, and pepper.
2. Warm the tortillas in a skillet or microwave according to package instructions.
3. Assemble tacos by placing a spoonful of quinoa and black bean mixture onto each tortilla.
4. Top with shredded lettuce, diced tomatoes, chopped fresh cilantro, and sliced avocado.
5. To make the Greek yogurt sauce, combine Greek yogurt, lime juice, chopped fresh cilantro, salt, and pepper in a small bowl.
6. Drizzle Greek yogurt sauce over the tacos.
7. Serve quinoa and black bean tacos immediately.

Nutrition Facts (per serving, 2 tacos):

- Calories: 350
- Carbohydrates: 45g
- Protein: 15g
- Fat: 15g

100. Chicken and Broccoli Cauliflower Rice Casserole

Prep.Time: 20 min

Cook Time: 30 min

Serving: 6

Beverage pairing: Green Tea

Ingredients:

- 2 cups cooked chicken breast, shredded
- 4 cups cauliflower rice
- 2 cups broccoli florets, chopped
- 1 onion, diced
- 2 cloves garlic, minced
- 1 cup shredded cheddar cheese
- 1 cup Greek yogurt
- 1/4 cup grated Parmesan cheese
- 1 teaspoon dried thyme
- Salt and pepper to taste
- Olive oil for cooking

Preparation:

1. Preheat oven to 375°F (190°C). Grease a 9x13-inch baking dish.
2. Heat olive oil in a skillet over medium heat. Add diced onion and minced garlic. Sauté until onions are translucent. Add chopped broccoli florets to the skillet and cook until slightly softened.
3. In a large bowl, combine cooked chicken breast, cauliflower rice, cooked broccoli mixture, shredded cheddar cheese, Greek yogurt, grated Parmesan cheese, dried thyme, salt, and pepper. Mix until well combined. Transfer the mixture to the prepared baking dish and spread it out evenly.
4. Bake in the preheated oven for 25-30 minutes, or until the top is golden brown and bubbly.
5. Remove from the oven and let it cool for a few minutes before serving.
6. Serve chicken and broccoli cauliflower rice casserole hot.

Nutrition Facts (per serving):

- Calories: 300
- Carbohydrates: 10g
- Protein: 30g
- Fat: 15g

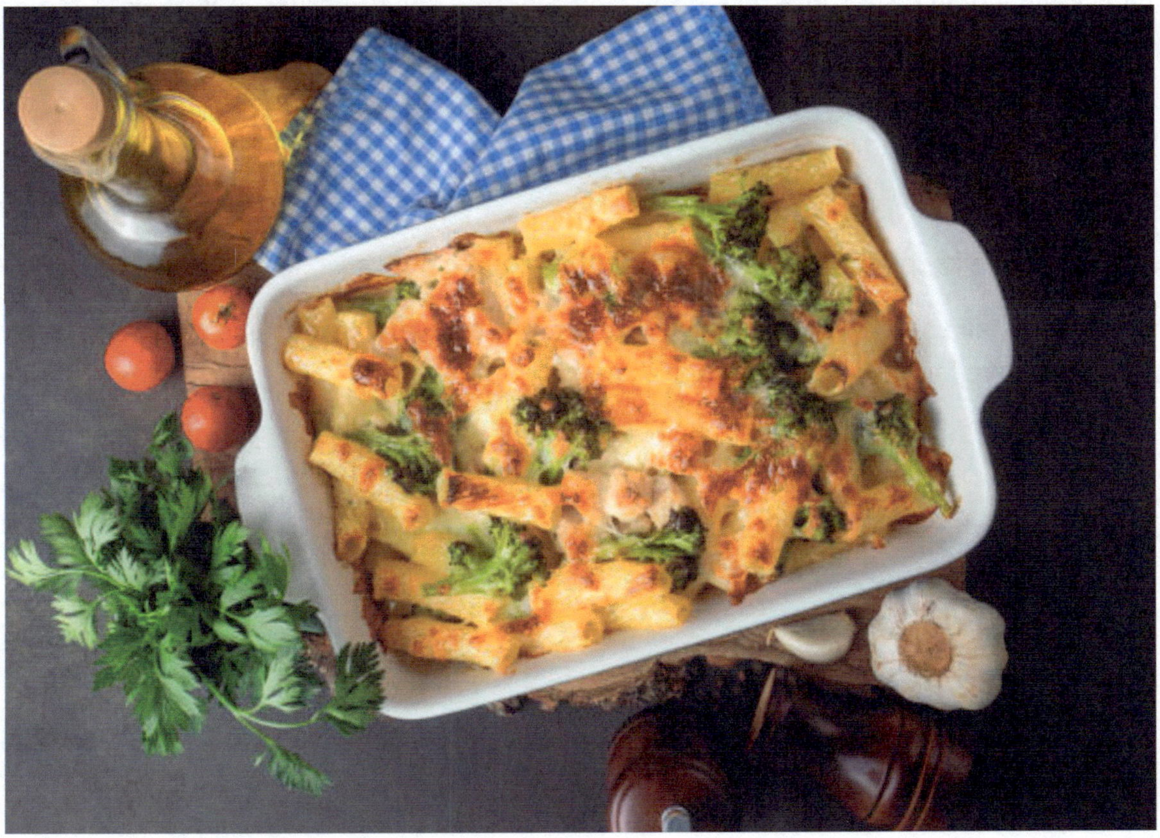

Sharing Your Culinary Journey

Now that you've mastered the art of creating delicious, diabetes-friendly meals, it's time to share your newfound culinary wisdom with others who are on the same path. By leaving your honest review of the "Type 2 Diabetes Cookbook: Beginner's Quick & Easy Recipes for Delicious Diabetes Diets" by Lily Anders on Amazon, you'll guide fellow food enthusiasts to a resource that can transform their dining table and health.

Your insights and experiences are invaluable, offering a beacon to those navigating their diet amidst diabetes. Whether it was a specific recipe that became your go-to, a tip that changed how you approach cooking, or the overall ease and enjoyment you found in these pages, your feedback is a gift that keeps on giving.

Thank you for contributing to a community of knowledge and support. The journey towards healthy eating and diabetes management thrives on shared discoveries and successes. By passing on your review, you're not just recommending a book—you're enriching lives with the joy of cooking and the empowerment of dietary control.

>>> Click Below to leave your review on Amazon <<<

https://www.amazon.com/dp/1963939352

Together, we're keeping the passion for healthy, joyful eating alive, one review at a time. Your support makes all the difference, not just to us, but to every reader and cook who seeks to balance their love for food with their health needs.

- With heartfelt thanks,

Lily Anders

Conclusion

In conclusion, this book transcends the traditional approach to managing diabetes through diet alone, offering a comprehensive guide that empowers individuals with diabetes to navigate their condition with knowledge and precision. Through 300 carefully crafted recipes, we explore the importance of balancing nutrient intake and the vital role of consistent meal planning. Each recipe is not just a set of instructions but a building block towards a healthier life, tailored to the unique needs of those managing diabetes.

As we close this journey of understanding and adaptation, remember that managing diabetes is not just about adhering to dietary restrictions or grappling with numbers—it is about reclaiming control of your health and life. These recipes are designed not only to meet specific nutritional needs but also to delight the palate, proving that a diabetes-conscious diet can be as delicious as it is nutritious.

Embrace these culinary tools as your allies in the pursuit of wellness. Let each meal enrich your body and spirit, and may the knowledge contained in this book guide you toward a balanced, joyful, and healthy life with diabetes. Here's to finding pleasure in every bite and strength in every challenge. Cheers to your health and happiness on this flavorful journey!

Made in United States
Cleveland, OH
05 November 2026

47768324R00071